A Happy End of Life

Living Well after 80

Wolfgang Berg and Jay Pomerantz

Thoughts, Experiences, and Research
About the last twenty Years of your Life

Cover Photo:
Marianna Hagan, with her five Gold Medals at the National Senior Olympics Swimming Competition in the age bracket 90 and over.

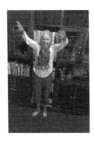

About this book

> The last years of your life can be downright ugly.
> But nothing is so bad that it could not get worse.
> Or better.
> The difference is small.
> You can provide the direction, up or down.
> This book will help making the "the last score" pleasant.

We discuss climate change and the living conditions of 100 and 200 years in the future, but how about our living conditions in 20 or 40 years? Our present actions will have dramatic consequences for our own lives over 80.

This book should make 40-year-olds think and plan about their future, while it is still time to actually do something about it with ease and little cost.

And those at age 80 will find solutions and encouragement for a happy last quintile.

This book is written in two parts: "The Aging Body" derives from the personal life experiences of Wolfgang Berg, an 84-year-old. He brings observations from high-level amateur sports and personal stories of encounters with people living all over the world. He engages with older people who live on remote islands, mountain outposts, and next door in urban spaces. He tells us of his studies of geriatrics, nutrition, wellness, and financial planning. He interviews retirees in nursing homes and studies elderly folks for consumer and marketing research purposes. He shares his thoughts on living a long, happy, and healthy life.

By contrast, the second part "The Aging Brain" by Jay M Pomerantz, MD, describes findings from neuroscience that increase the odds for people to enjoy the last quintile of life in health and happiness. It is the result of 50 years of psychiatric practice as well as research and teaching about the aging brain.

The two parts reinforce each other. The result is an inspirational, practical, and scientific guide to health and happiness towards the end of life.

Table of Contents

About this book 3

Mind and Body. Horse and Carriage. 9

Part I: The Aging Body 12

1.   What is Life? 13
2.   Life Expectancy 17
3.   What is Aging? 20
   - a) The Biological Aging Process 21
   - b) The Culture of Aging 26
   - c) Appearances: Looking Old 30
   - d) Don't Die Prematurely 32
4.   Staying Fit Mentally and Physically 38
5.   You are what you eat 42
   - a) You are a Chemical Factory: Metabolism 44
   - b) Naked on the Scale 45
   - c) You Are Still In The Stone Age 47
6.   Health 50
   - a) Absence of Illness? 50
   - b) Gamble With Your Life – And Win 52
   - c) The Living Cell 54
   - d) Health Care 58
7.   Care and Nursing homes 60
   - a) Search and Plan Well 60
   - b) Good Company 61
   - c) The Cost of Care 63

8.	Money	68
9.	Life in Retirement	74
10.	Happiness	75
a)	The Happiest Moments in My Life	75
b)	The Myth of Happiness	76
c)	Feeling Happy	78
d)	Status	79
e)	Self- Esteem	81
f)	The Chemistry of Happiness	83
g)	Future and Present Happiness	85
h)	Happy and Unhappy People	86
i)	Expectations	88
j)	Unhappiness and Depression	91
k)	Tragedy and Other Problems	93
11.	Religion	98
12.	Facing the End	101
13.	The End	105
Further Reading		107

Part II: the Aging Brain 108

1.	The Brain of a Sea Slug	111
2.	The Memory of a Taxi Driver	113
3.	Muscle Memory	114
4.	Teaching an Old Dog New Tricks	115
5.	Old Mice Getting Younger	116
6.	Dementia	117
7.	Dementia Prevalence by Age Groups	119
8.	Preventing Dementia?	120

9.	The Nun Study	122
10.	Physical Exercise	124
11.	The Spark Plugs in our Brain	126
12.	Keeping the Brain Young	128
13.	The Importance of Sleep	130
14.	Telomeres	132
15.	Stress	135
16.	Acute Stress	136
17.	Chronic Stress	138
18.	Major Depression	139
19.	Chronic Stress and Cardiovascular Disease	141
20.	Emotional Resilience	143
21.	The Monkey's Mothering Attachment	146
22.	Human Attachment	148
23.	Maternal Deprivation	149
24.	Chronic Stress versus Emotional Resilience	150
25.	Characteristics of Resilient Individuals	151
26.	A Third-World Mental Hospital	152
27.	Are the Old Happier than the Young?	157
28.	The Future: Longevity and Anti-Aging Research	161

About the Authors 163
  Wolfgang Berg 163
  Jay M. Pomerantz, M.D. 164

End Notes   165

Mind and Body. Horse and Carriage.

This book intends to answer the question: How can you increase the odds of making the latter years of your life pleasant and not miserable? It also suggests that you may possibly live longer and more healthfully.

We divided this book into two parts. The traditional definition of life is the life of the body as we see and experience it. So, the first part focuses on the aging body. That, however, is incomplete. People have known for thousands of years that life involves both mind and body. The Roman and Greek philosophy of a healthy life was *"Mens sana in corpore sano,"* or "A healthy mind in a healthy body." Both mind and body are also acknowledged in a saying that originated somewhere in middle-ages Germany, *"Essen und Trinken hält Leib und Seele zusammen,"* meaning "eating and drinking keeps body and soul together."

So, back to the first part of the book. It is primarily the observation of people and experiences of one of the authors, Wolfgang Berg, alive and kicking at 84.

With friends dying around me, I ask, "What's keeping me young?" Well, I never had the intention of early suicide, lived a healthy life style because I was competitive in sports, although not terribly talented, and I met friends like the other author, Jay Pomerantz, from whom I learned a lot about life and death as science sees it today. I did a lot of research: not medical research, but research of consumers about behavior and preferences. I travelled to many different countries in Europe, North and South America, Japan and China. I also sailed to remote islands. By the way, Dominica in the Caribbean has more people over 100 years of age per capita than almost anywhere else.

Besides all that, I had dreams. I was pursuing a dream to save the world. That's nonsense of course. Many times, I discussed with friends and sailors, sitting at night on a sailboat under millions of stars, how to improve the world. My supposition was that nobody would listen to me. Until, one day a friend said, "Wolfgang, what's your secret? Why don't you write about it?"

So, what is it? Nutrition? Sports? Meditation? Having a purpose or a goal? I just learned that people with a life purpose live significantly longer. Well, my goal is to win the national tennis championship for 100-year-olds. I am on my way and working at it, enjoying every year I get older. Retirement? Forget it.

So, I started to write things down, read studies, and interview people, young and old. Marianna, my neighbor, has a pacemaker and has had several heart operations, but she keeps swimming. She just won her 5th gold medal in the Senior Olympics at 93. Risky? "Yes, but if I die, it should be in a race." Perhaps, with this book, I can make a difference; writing this book might offer ideas and help for others. Another purpose for my life!

A recent study found that tennis leads all sports in how long its participants stay alive. The Copenhagen City Heart Study examined people over a 25-year period and evaluated improvements in life expectancy through participation in various sports and leisure-time activities. In total, 8,577 participants were examined for all causes of mortality between 1991 and 2017. Tennis topped the charts for potential life-expectancy gains with results suggesting as many as 9.7 years could be added to an individual's existence.

This is 3.5 years more than its nearest competitor, badminton, the playing of which has been found to increase life expectancy by 6.2 years, with soccer having the potential to add 4.7 years and cycling, 3.7 years.

Swimming was found to boost life expectancy rates by 3.4 years, jogging by 3.2 years, calisthenics by 3.1 years, and health club activities by 1.5 years.

A further conclusion of the study suggests that leisure-time sports which involve greater levels of *social interaction* are associated with higher levels of longevity.[1]

Maybe my discussions with tennis friends about how to improve the world could be part of my secret. This takes me to Jay Pomerantz, another tennis player over 80 and in good health.

Jay opened my eyes beyond the aging body, to the aging brain. He keeps up with advances in neuroscience.

His career in psychiatry/neuroscience started after medical school with a Peace Corps volunteer job at a mental hospital in Panama that would be better described as a mental prison. That experience re-directed his career. He wrote Part II, "The Aging Brain."

Most surprising for our readers will be the revelation that the two-way interaction our brain is having with our bodies and environment can affect the brain's structure, function, and health. The brain is "plastic," constantly changing shape and capacity throughout life. This information brings us as close as ever to the mysterious Fountain of Youth. But instead of buying a glass of that water in St. Augustine, Florida, the reader will drink a bit of wisdom in this book, which not only costs less but is more likely to have a better effect.

Part I: The Aging Body

1. What is Life?

The first rule for a pleasant end is to understand the reality of life:

> *The purpose of our lives is to be happy.*
> *- Tenzin Gyatso, the 14th Dalai Lama*
>
> *The purpose of human life is to serve, and to show compassion and the will to help others.*
> *- Albert Schweitzer*
>
> *Cogito ergo sum (I think, therefore I am).*
> *- Descartes*
>
> *The meaning of life is to give life meaning.*
> *- Viktor E. Frankl*

"Everything comes to an end," says Buddha. "Not true," says the physicist, "every action causes a reaction, nothing ever ends."

But when I am dead, I am dead. Period. "That depends," says the biologist, "on how you define life." Your individual life really does not matter. What matters is the life of the species. You are only a cell that keeps the species alive. Cells are created and die. It is analogous to leaves that fall and decay, but the tree stays alive. Birth and death are designed for the survival of the species. So, don't cry if you have done your job.

Imagine what would happen if humans could survive 1000 years and the reproductive cycle took 500 years. Evolution would take twenty times longer. Humanoids with fur and long fingers living in trees would have found it hard to survive in the savannah when the climate changed and much of the rainforest disappeared. Our direct ancestors would have become extinct right then. In fact, many other types of humanoids did become extinct, but Lucy, the world's most famous early human ancestor, survived, since her folks adapted fast enough, meaning they reproduced fast and died fast.

There were numerous climate changes in the last two million years, and each time, humans adapted relatively quickly. They lost the fur, walked upright, developed a darker skin to protect from the intense sun, and made fire at night.

Then, during the last major drought, one hundred thousand years ago, they moved north along the Nile. They followed migrating herds of game north to regions with little sun. Since their bodies needed Vitamin D, which is created when sun rays interact with the skin, the northerners dropped the dark skin protection.

Every generation experiences multiple random mutations in their DNA. By chance, some of the changes may prove beneficial in adapting to a changed environment. "Survival of the fittest," when combined with relatively short life span and regeneration periods, helps a species adapt to new conditions. Fruit flies recreate in two days; some bacteria double in twenty minutes. We can't compete with that. Yet, extreme longevity, as much as people desire it, is not in the best interest of the human species. Dinosaurs and mammoths went extinct in part because each individual lived too long, and the species could not adapt to a changed climate.

After hunting large animals into scarcity, humans invented agriculture and adapted to a new lifestyle. A more recent adaptation was overcoming lactose intolerance to be able to digest cows' milk. Now, some of us are trying to adapt to junk food. That doesn't seem to be going particularly well. The short duration that constitutes an individual life may be divided into five parts of twenty years each:

1. Growing up to twenty.
2. Mating and reproduction from twenty to forty.
3. Working hard for family and society from forty to sixty.
4. Supporting grandchildren with care and wisdom from sixty to eighty.
5. After that you are free to goof off, play, and do whatever you like, travel to foreign countries and eventually to heaven. This last period is what we are talking about: 80 to whenever.

We all know that life is finite. Even if science finds a way to extend it, life will still be finite. So, in this book, we are not focusing on extending life. The question is, how can we make this final period pleasant?

But adding "pleasant" into the discussion is tricky. Indeed, that is the rationale for some to shorten their lives. The most popular "suicide" is suicide for pleasure. Drugs, alcohol, smoking, junk food, or even lying on the couch all day are known to be unhealthy, but "Hell, you only live once." It's not just death for pleasure; also quite popular is dying due to misinformation, lifestyle, economics, environment, or accidents.

We aim to shed light on these issues and hopefully nudge others to see it the way we do. Short-term pleasure has its long-term consequences. What is a pleasant old age? Being healthy and rich?

First, it would be nice not to run out of money just because one happens to live five years longer than expected. Wouldn't it be a good idea to think about that before it happens, when you still have income?

Second, life is much more pleasant without pains and disabilities. Take a look at older folks and pick your idol. At what age did they start living a long, happy life? Or ask an old person in pain if she or he is enjoying life. Was smoking, drinking, overeating, and never exercising worth a shorter life? I asked a few and everyone said "I should have…" I also heard young people say, "You only live once; I rather enjoy life." That may be okay, if you are having fun and then die. But with the help of modern medicine, people live longer, sometimes to the age of regret.

Everybody wishes to have a long life, but few make a decision to have a *pleasant* long life. It is a decision for a lifestyle.

Some who have sinned against life may be lucky if a serious illness strikes and gets them back on the right track when there still is time. And lucky are those young oddballs, who dared to be different, revolting against social pressure and did not use drugs when all others did. It's a bit late to start living healthy at eighty, but it is never completely too late and never too early.

People wish to have a long life, but what is life? Who am I? Am I a body with a head, arms, and legs that I want to be in good operating condition forever? Is it eyes that see, ears that listen, tongues that taste, feelings, a brain with memories that I want to keep alive? Or is it the chemical factory of a billion cells that produce 75,000 enzymes and hormones that make us love, fear, freeze, sweat, and struggle to stay alive? Look in a mirror, naked, smile at yourself, and ask: Who am I? What am I?

There are many answers to these questions. For what it is worth, I will provide my thoughts. Your conscious existence is not you, or not determined by you, but by society. Your friends, your community, colleagues, club members, customers, doctors, parents, family members. In other words, the world around you defines you. The world positions you relative to all other people. You have a status and belong. Look at wolves, whales, geese or bees. The worst that can happen is your wolf family expels you. I saw a documentary where a lone wolf tried to join another group and was killed. A group of terrorists brainwashes a suicide bomber to sacrifice his life. He would help his family; he would save the world and go to heaven. That's not you. Or is it? You dress yourself to be approved, you grow a lawn instead tomatoes, so your neighbors approve of you, and you shop for weeks to get the right car for your personality. Your house, your job, and your hobbies define you. Striving for status is one of the basic biological motivations. To preserve status, or some call it honor, many people actually sacrifice their physical existence. And if, in the final years of your physical life, you can manage to be well-liked, respected, and loved, if you are conscious of all the good things you did for the world and for your family, you will be happy, even with pain, even when things come to an end. With that fulfilment, you will continue to exist even after your heart stops beating.

Physical birth and death are essential life functions of all species. Living the last twenty years in happy fulfilment requires you to understand your role as a productive human life from beginning to end.

Understanding the reality of life does not make you fearless of death. Fear is a natural life protector. But understanding life will prevent you from panicking and making wrong or no decisions. You will face the inevitable with courage and in comfort.

2. Life Expectancy

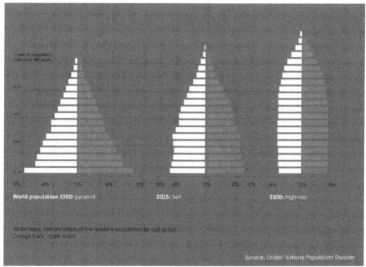

Population Age Pyramid 1950 to 2100

Humans will live longer. Instead of younger people dying gradually at all ages, which is represented by the typical pyramid shape on the left, people will live to 100 at the end of this century, but then die relatively abruptly between 80 and 100, which is the pyramid on the right.

How long will you live? Begin by testing your life expectancy. Make sure you don't enter advertising scams or websites that capture your personal data before they respond. Below are three websites that I have tried. The more questions they ask, the better the results:

http://media.nmfn.com/tnetwork/lifespan/#0

http://www.worldlifeexpectancy.com/life-expectancy-test

https://www.livingto100.com/users

Let's say your life expectancy is between 84 and 104. If you are 60, you have between 24 and 34 years to live. That may give you enough time to make some preparations. I don't mean reserving a cemetery plot. I mean, time to make financial plans and plans for feeling great and having affordable care when you need it. If you are 80 and in good health, you may live between eight and 24 more years.

The life expectancy test will give you a life span and also recommendations for a lifestyle that extends your life and keeps you fit and healthy. However, you know yourself better. You are not a statistical average but an individual that learns and has the ability to make intelligent decisions each day.

Most effective, but not covered in any test, is your vision of yourself and your future. Your vision of yourself determines your way of life. The best improvement in my whole life was a one-week course in meditation. Prayer is certainly also a way of self-programming. Meditation empowers your subconscious to find solutions for just about everything, including financial, business, relationship, and health problems.

The statistical life prediction websites will not give you a best case or worst-case scenario about the end game. That's something you must draw up yourself.

A good ending could be this: You stay healthy, fit, and accident-free, driving a car safely and living in your own home until age 95. From 95 to 100, you hire daytime assistance for home and garden, and perhaps some therapist visits you twice a week. You use Uber and senior care transportation by your township and participate in available senior programs. From 100 to 105, you order all meals for home delivery online, get help in therapy and daily care at home, enjoy support by family members, and on one hot day, during a little too much exercise, you experience a heart attack, and that's it.

My friend Milton just passed away at age 104. Three years ago, he entered a luxury nursing home. Unfortunately, his pinochle game had suffered due to a stroke at age 99, but generally he had been in good health to the end. There is only one problem with getting that old: It costs more.

A worst-case scenario health wise may be financially your best case, since you pass away earlier. At 85, you may have a minor accident at home with a head injury. The result, however, is not so minor. Now there are difficulties with memory, mobility, hearing and vision, and bowels. While hospitalized, you pass out. That happened to my grandmother. She was a bit overweight and never participated in any exercise except short walks with her dog. She was a good cook and a good homemaker. She was fixing the old-fashioned overhead toilet tank when the toilet lid slid and she fell, hitting her head on the tiles. She died three months later.

At age 40, and even at 60, it is easy to make changes in your lifestyle. At 70, it should be your highest priority to make plans and take action preparing for the last twenty years. At 80, most people are so afraid of death that they don't even want to think about an exit plan. I hope that this book will help you work towards a desirable scenario.

3. What is Aging?

You can be run over by a drunken driver tomorrow and die. However, according to statistics, you will live another 20 years, perhaps 15 or even 23. You have determined a range of years to live with best case and worst-case scenarios. The life expectancy test has given you hints for extending your life, such as four extra years by eating three portions of fruits and vegetables a day. One website told me to drink a glass or two of wine a day (I don't touch alcohol). I assume that website was sponsored by the wine industry.

Most living species don't want to die. But I believe most animals know when life is over, and they just die. My neighbor's old cat went away one day and never came back. But most civilized humans are obsessed with extending life at all cost. For what? Do you really have to finish a job, a project, or a mission? Are you required by your family or your bank to live 4 ½ years longer?

We will deal with those questions, but the main purpose of this book is not to extend life. It is to enjoy the life that you are given, whether it is the next month or the next 25 years

a) The Biological Aging Process

We can observe aging but know little about how it works. The first signs of getting old may be gray hair, followed by a loss of fertility and loss of hair, then far-sightedness and some arthritis. Our strength and endurance weakens. We have hearing problems, then memory problems, and at age 85 to 90, approximately 30-40 percent of us get Alzheimer's or another form of dementia. Arteriosclerosis causes heart attacks or a stroke, possible brain damage, organ failures, and finally death. An old person has wrinkles and a bent posture, a squeaky voice and walks with uncertain little steps.

What are the reasons for all this? One explanation is damage caused by wear and tear. Cartilage wears off, skin dries out, vertebral discs shrink, and deposits of fat, toxic proteins, and calcium damage a variety of organs.

Another explanation is that aging is programmed into our DNA. Specific genes may cause aging by slowing growth of new cells, and the result is that organs begin to fail, and the body looks and functions differently, like that of an old person.

Several studies have found that physical and mental exercise, a healthy diet, sufficient sleep, and social interaction correlate with a healthy and long life. Dr. Robert Butler, the first director of the National Institute on Aging, found that an ability to *define your life's meaning adds to your life expectancy*. Individuals who expressed a clear goal in life—something to get up for in the morning, something that made a difference—lived longer and were sharper than those who did not.

While most studies show correlations, some recent research suggests a direct relationship between aging and our DNA. The ends of our chromosomes, called telomeres, keep DNA vital and healthy until they shorten with age. Several factors directly affect the length of telomeres. The strongest factor is chronic mental stress. Part II of this book, "The Aging Brain," explains how the aging brain is particularly vulnerable but can also develop resilience.

A recent study in Current Biology[2] documents that small DNA mutations significantly increase biological age[3]. Data from over a thousand older adults showed that the 6 percent of the population with physical mutations had a biological age four years older than the participants without the mutations. The group with the acquired mutations had an increase in age-related diseases such as blood cancers, heart disease, and Alzheimer's.

Perhaps more relevant is that not only aging damages DNA, but chronic inflammation does as well. When the immune system goes into a hypervigilant state, it produces reactive oxygen and nitrogen compounds to attack bacteria or other toxic or hostile substance that cause diseases, but these chemicals (including hydrogen peroxide, nitric oxide, and hypochlorous acid) can also damage the body's own biomolecules, including DNA.

The question then arises about how to control or decrease chronic inflammation. One possible way is to increase the intake of anti-inflammatory foods. In the study[4] of 68,273 Swedish men and women aged 45 to 83 who were followed for 16 years, participants who most closely followed an anti-inflammatory diet had an 18 percent lower risk of all-cause mortality, a 20 percent lower risk of cardiovascular mortality, and a 13 percent lower risk of cancer mortality when compared with those who followed the diet to a lesser degree.

Anti-inflammatory foods consist of fruits and vegetables, tea, coffee, whole grain bread, breakfast cereal, low-fat cheese, olive oil and canola oil, nuts, chocolate, and moderate amounts of red wine and beer. Pro-inflammatory foods include unprocessed and processed red meat, organ meats, chips, and soft-drink beverages.

In order to further understand the biological process of aging, we have to dig down into the cells of our body. Cells multiply and die continuously. They can get sick and malfunction. All cells experience changes with aging. They become larger and are less able to divide and multiply. Among other changes, there is an increase in pigments and fatty substances inside the cell. Cell membranes become less efficient in taking in oxygen and nutrients or removing carbon dioxide and other metabolic products.

Living tissue is made up of similar cells which come together to perform particular functions. In turn, the different kinds of tissues come together to form organs. Thus, all of our organs are aging and gradually becoming less functional over time. Therefore, as you grow older, you will have changes throughout your body, including changes in enzyme and hormone production, immunity, skin, sleep, bones, muscles, joints, breasts, face, reproductive organs, heart and blood vessels, kidneys, lungs, brain, and nervous system.

Let's use the heart as an example. With increasing age, all the structures of the heart become more rigid. The muscles of the left ventricle get thicker, the heart may increase slightly in size, and the volume of the left ventricle may decline. As a result, the heart may both fill and empty more slowly, thus putting less blood into circulation. The increase in one's heart rate and cardiac output in response to physical activity is also diminished, and one's maximum heart rate declines. The drop in maximum heart rate appears to be greater than average in sedentary individuals and in those with overt cardiovascular disease. What we are talking about here is not disease, but normal loss of function with increasing age.

Most people do not notice the various losses of vital functions over time because it is slow, and there is spare capacity. A nice example is kidney function. One only needs 25 percent of maximal kidney function to sustain life well.

The problem is that when an organ with diminished capacity is worked harder than usual, it may not be able to increase function. Most commonly, an illness will show the compromised organ function. For example, a simple urinary tract infection will throw a compromised kidney into renal failure, whereas it will not affect the ability of a well-functioning kidney to excrete waste products.

The aging process affects all organs, so the skin of old people is thinner, bruises more easily, and older people feel the cold more than younger folks. Joints deteriorate and cause inflammation and pain which we call arthritis. Lungs get stiff, and the capacity for strenuous exercise diminishes with age. Our brains lose neurons and synapses, and forgetfulness is common in old age. On and on.

Despite this rather depressing picture of cellular, tissue, and organ function in old age, all is not lost. The measures we are advocating in this book may decrease the powerful effects of organ aging. Let's take an easily measured and well-researched topic: lung function. The most widely used measure of maximal functional capacity is peak oxygen consumption (VO_2), which is measured on a treadmill or cycle ergometer. In cross-sectional studies, peak VO_2 typically declines eight to ten percent per age decade in healthy men and women. Recent long-term studies have even shown declines in peak VO_2 of 20-25 percent per decade in healthy elders older than 70 years. On the other hand, the peak VO_2 in distance runners aged 60-80 years was 30 to 40 percent higher than nontrained but active age-peers in the Baltimore Longitudinal Study of Aging (BLSA); in fact, their aerobic capacity was similar to that of BLSA participants 2-3 decades younger. [5] [6]

Although not yet yielding specific advice, there is a new player in the aging space: epigenetics. While traditional genetics describes the way the DNA sequences in our genes are passed from one generation to the next, epigenetics determines which of our genes are switched-on, or "expressed." Epigenetics explains how our upbringing, diet, and current internal and external environment affects which of the 20,000+ genes are switched on and off in the various cells of the body. What you eat, where you live, who you interact with, when you sleep, how you exercise— all of these can eventually cause chemical modifications around the genes (epigenetic changes) that will turn those genes on or off over time. Furthermore, the instability of the epigenome seems to increase with age, adversely affecting cellular function and stress resistance.[7]

Therefore, understanding age-dependent epigenomic changes should eventually yield insights into how aging begins and progresses as well as leading to the development of new therapeutics that delay or even reverse aging and age-related diseases.

The above discussion and evidence suggest ways for prolonging a healthy life, but ever since the fountain of youth that Ponce de Leon thought of having discovered, commercialism has sold pills for extending life, and people are willing to try anything with such promises. While science makes great advances, we have to be more cautious about such claims. I keep seeing commercials on television for Prevagen with the claim that it improves short term memory by 25 percent. Indeed, the sales of supplements to improve memory are a three-billion-dollar (2016) business. And here is the evidence or lack thereof:

An AARP sponsored study on brain health by an independent body of top scientists, doctors, scholars, and policy experts found that "scientific evidence does not support the use of any supplement to prevent, slow, reverse or stop cognitive decline or dementia or other related neurological disease such as Alzheimer's"[8].

While we are at it, what is the evidence that red wine is helpful in warding off heart disease, thereby increase longevity? For starters, there is the "French Paradox," wherein the French have relatively low rates of heart disease, even though their diet is high in saturated fats such as butter and cheese. Indeed, red wine is high in resveratrol, which mimics dietary restriction, a known but difficult-to-practice longevity factor. The problem is that resveratrol is not very potent and also not very soluble in the human gut. You would have to drink a hundred to a thousand glasses of red wine daily to get an amount equivalent to the doses that improved health in mice![9]

b)   The Culture of Aging

We all observe how people grow up, become mature, then look older, become weaker, and finally pass away. This observation is common knowledge. The phases of aging are known to everyone in society, and our culture is structured around age.

Classification by age group is all around us. Adulthood starts with the drinking age, the voting age, and the privilege to serve in the military.

Then there is parenting and a job or professional career.

At 55, you are old. Employers want younger people.

Soon approaching is retirement age, defined in many different ways, but not by physical or mental ability.

There are senior communities for those 55 and over.

At 65, you have likely reached retirement.

Some form of social security was established in the 17th century, first by the English "Poor Law," also by trade unions, and in the newly founded United States in 1776. Later, a U.S. law established a support program for veterans and widows of the Civil War. Eventually, this became a military pension program. It was an attractive incentive to recruit soldiers. In Germany, the Prussian government introduced a pension program for state employees.

When the average life expectancy was 45 in 1840, such programs could be easily financed by taxation. Since most were dying early, there was no outcry for national pension plans for the general public.

A long-term trend of growing life expectancy started in 1870. This happened because of improving public health programs, especially safe drinking water and proper elimination of human waste. Better childbirth practices also saved many lives. Yet, in 1900, life expectancy in the United States was still approximately 47.

The American Social Security Program was established in 1935, when life expectancy was around 60. After a typical wartime decrease of life expectancy, it shot up after World War II. From then on, antibiotics and many other medications extended the life of older people.

Presently, the life expectancy is around 80 years with a yearly growth trend of three months per year over the last 40 years. This would lead to an average life expectancy of 95 in the year 2050.

Nearly 30 percent of the US population is over 55 years old, which is a strong senior voting base supporting social security and tax-advantaged pension plans. Soon, retirees will outnumber workers. Will we vote for a faster way to bankruptcy or for a radical overhaul of our political system that produces more value for all? Individually, the challenge is to prepare for a reduction of benefits and increase of taxes.

There was a time when the few that made it to old age could be easily supported by the younger ones. The old were, in fact, a valuable asset. The elders were the wisest, the teachers, and the bearers of tradition and knowledge. Old women knew herbs and mushrooms, baking and cooking, cures for illnesses, and all about childbirth. Old men knew the migration of game, could read the clouds, could teach hunting, and could tell old stories about wars with enemies and about the history of their ancestors.

Today, wisdom comes from Google, Wikipedia, and television shows. Old people are thought to be not up to date with technology and fashion. Over 80, they are considered to be senile, though their money is appreciated to help out the younger generations.

Younger generations may even resent the well-meant advice of the elders. Therefore, old people often socialize with other old people, where they get mutual respect.

Since we are social beings, we are influenced by culture and society's classification. So, if you want to enjoy the last twenty years of your life, you have to be quietly rebellious. If you feel young and agile, you have to free yourself from the attitude of being old.

You have to be an outcast, a quiet revolutionary.

A sailing friend of mine has the attitude that life is going downhill from birth. He can't go sailing anymore with me since he says, "I am too old." On our last cruise through the Bahamas, we landed at an island and met a very old couple in a small resort. We engaged in the usual conversation. We went from "where are you from," to "Are you having a good vacation," and proceeded to "Mind me asking, how old are you?"

"I am 95," said the man. "I am 94," said the woman.

"And you still travel to the islands? What are you doing here?"

"We are building a house," said the man.

"A house?" asked my friend. "Do you have a good contractor?"

"No, we are building it ourselves."

It hit him like a bombshell. In my friend's mind, by defying "old age," you are some sort of odd ball. But you are not alone. You will find people who respect your experience and reinforce your positive thinking.

I often hear that old people complain about forgetting things. Think about what you forgot when you were twenty. If you dislike forgetfulness, keep a calendar in your pocket and write everything down. Are you making stupid mistakes and assuming those are the result of old age? How many dumb mistakes did you make when you were young?

Sixty percent of people over 60 have a loss in hearing. What did you say? A sure sign of old age. It might be time for a professional hearing evaluation and maybe a hearing aid.

Many people at 35 have back pain. But they don't attribute it to old age. At 70, however, you are prone to think it's your age. Medical professionals often perpetuate this myth. My great uncle developed pain in his left knee at age 95. He went to the doctor, who told him it was just a by-product of his advanced age. Whereupon, he asked the doctor if his right knee was younger than the left one, as he had no pain in that knee!

I had severe back pain at 35 to 40. Doctors told me to stop playing tennis. I wanted surgery but ended up with a prestigious surgeon who surprised me by saying he would not operate. Instead, he gave me a booklet with simple exercises. I never had back pain again. Now, at 84, I am a nationally ranked tennis player in my age group, and I enjoy getting older. I can't wait to get into the 90s, and my goal is to win the nationals for 100 and over, although this age bracket does not exist yet.

My neighbor, Marianna, whose picture is on the cover of this book, has severe heart problems. She should not be swimming at her age. However, she is training hard every day. She is over 90 and recently won five gold medals in the Senior Olympics. "When I die, I hope it's in a race." Now she is on her way to the Senior Olympics again.

c) Appearances: Looking Old

It is not only your own attitude that impacts you. It is also the attitude of others. I am talking about the reflection of your image from others back to you. It is a like looking in the mirror. What you see has an effect on you.

How do you create a positive image? Should you use cosmetics in an effort to look like twenty? Anybody can see it is fake and may think either you are a faker or disconnected from reality.

The first sign of a youthful appearance is body language. Psychology[10] has found that if you smile, you feel happy. And others will like you for your smile. You, in turn, feel good because they smile back.

Walk like a ballerina with a swinging pace; don't drag along. Wear cushioned shoes. Your best gym is the parking lot; walk with a fast pace from your car to the store.

Try to keep your shoulders straight with good posture.

Have a firm handshake.

Look people in the eye. Be confident that you are at least as good as they are but be respectful of others. Give others respect, and they will pay you back in kind. Your confidence will rise.

Take good care of your clothing. Don't overdress and don't wear out-of-style dresses, shirts, suits, or the tie that should have been donated decades ago. Dress elegantly, clean, sporty, and dynamic.

Get a haircut, trim your eyebrows and the hair in ears and nose. Get your teeth fixed.

If you are in the sun a lot, you may have a nice tan, but if you don't wear sun lotion, your skin will certainly wrinkle, and you will be raising the risk for skin cancer, including melanomas. Soap washes away the skin's natural protection. Too frequent use of soap and shampoo is sometimes a problem. Using moisturizing skin cream often works miracles

Get a large brush with soft rubberized bristles and brush your whole body from top to bottom every morning and evening. Your skin is a very important organ and massaging it frequently will keep it alive and also improve blood circulation.

Try speaking loudly and clearly, with better pronunciation than today's teenagers. Your language should be friendly, meaningful, cultivated, but not overdone. Listening carefully and responding to what others say is more important than how much you say yourself.

Good communication is extremely important. If you don't hear well, your brain will get used to not understanding and reduce incoming messages to just sounds without meaning. You will not notice it at first, but it will damage your relationships. As I said before, wearing a hearing aid is considered a sign of old age, but the consequences of not wearing one are worse.

Think about not interrupting people and keeping your life stories short. You have been alive and had many experiences, but not everyone is interested in hearing all of them. Similarly, if you always talk about diseases and your health problems, people may find you depressing and even avoid you. Try talking more about positive things. You may even cheer yourself up!

d) Don't Die Prematurely

The Leading Causes of Death in 65+ Year-Olds Might Surprise You:[11]

#1: Heart Disease

Heart disease continues to be the top cause of death in older individuals. There has been some decrease due to widespread use of medication to lower cholesterol and blood pressure in affected individuals. Procedures to stent or bypass blocked coronary arteries have helped as well. Better and less intrusive surgery for heart valve disease has also helped. The Communicable Disease Center documents that 80 percent of heart disease deaths are attributable to lifestyle factors. Thus, changes in diet, activity, health management, etc. could prevent many deaths, and that is the point of much of this book.

#2: Cancer

As people live longer, cancer risk increases. Smoking and high alcohol intake correlate with an increase risk. Cancer is now much better treated than before with measures to strengthen the body's immune system now rendering some of the toxic chemotherapies obsolete. There are also preventative strategies to catch the disease early before it has spread. Periodic mammography, colonoscopy, and dermatologist visits for suspicious skin changes are several of the most important measures.

#3: Chronic Lower Respiratory Diseases

Chronic obstructive pulmonary disease (COPD) is often related to smoking or environmental causes. It tends to be a chronic illness that can be managed with various therapies. These include bronchodilator medications, inhalers, steroids, oxygen therapy, and pulmonary rehabilitation. Additionally, patients with COPD must carefully manage exacerbations and respiratory infections. This is where the condition can turn from chronic to fatal. Pulmonary rehabilitation involves exercise training, which strengthens the lungs and boosts immunity. Lack of activity makes pneumonia and other lung infections more likely. A yearly flu shot, although it varies in effectiveness from year to year, is a great investment. Not only is the incidence of flu decreased, but when individuals get sick, the illness tends to be less severe. For example, a 2017 study[12] showed that flu vaccination reduced deaths, intensive care unit (ICU) admissions, ICU length of stay, and overall duration of hospitalization among hospitalized flu patients. The observed benefits were greatest among people 65 years of age and older.

#4 Cerebrovascular Disease

The preventive strategies for heart disease apply equally to prevent cerebrovascular disease. Controlling both cholesterol and high blood pressure are paramount. Surgery is sometimes useful to bypass blocked large vessels supplying the brain. A yearly checkup with your physician will include attention to warning signs and checking for murmurs in the large blood vessels that pass through the neck region.

#5 Dementia Including Alzheimer's Disease

Please see Part II of this book for an extensive discussion of possible causes of dementia and ways to slow or possibly prevent this very difficult problem

#6 Diabetes

Elders with diabetes are prone to all kinds of potentially fatal health issues. Circulation and the immune system problems are common. It's essential for anyone with diabetes to monitor these concerns along with blood sugar levels and key vital signs. Even minor injuries can become fatal for a diabetic, and they may go unnoticed due to circulation problems and nerve damage. Thus, home safety is of utmost importance. Of course, the diabetic person also needs good nutritional support and proper medication management.

#7 Injuries

Deaths from unintentional injuries (accidents) were responsible for 2 percent, or about 34,000 deaths, in 2002 among people 65 years of age and older. Falls accounted for 55 percent of this total. Interestingly, mortality from accidents is almost twice as high among older men as women. Falls, motor vehicle crashes, suffocation, and burns account for most of the unintentional injury deaths among older persons.

Other studies[13] have shown that in the individuals over 80, functional limitations may be better at predicting further longevity than chronic medical conditions. Functional limitations include the capacity to perform five activities of daily living (bathing, dressing, eating, transferring in and out of bed, and toileting) and five instrumental activities of daily living (shopping, preparing meals, using the telephone, managing medications, and managing finances), and walking.

I have a particular respect for accidents, so I would like to address this topic more fully and personally.

Accidents are by definition unexpected. However, you can anticipate and avoid dangers that lead to accidents. Insurance companies define accidents precisely, and so could you. Accidents are not a result of old age. In fact, young people have more car accidents than older people. You have experience.

It is said that older people have a balance problem. True or not, it is always a good idea to stand on one leg when brushing your teeth. I like mountain hiking on narrow trails (within limits), and I even practice. When I walk on easy trails, I make it a habit to balance on ridges in the grass or dirt, and sometimes I walk on the curb.

Rugs and runners tend to skid. Wet tiles are a hazard. Slippery shoes are a deadly sin. Have salt, a snow shovel, and a hot water hose to de-ice your way to the car and your driveway. A rubber mat can help prevent slips and falls in the shower and bathtub. Your basement stairs are another concern. Do you have slip-proof rubber pads on the steps and side rails to prevent a fall? In fact, it is a good idea to have hand rails installed at any possibly dangerous spot around the house or apartment.

You may save a lot of money by doing repairs yourself, but wear safety glasses where sand or dust may get in your eyes. Just as obviously, wear gloves when painting and cleaning.

Secure tools, cords, and things in storage or safely on shelves. A friend just injured his arm when an object in his cluttered garage fell on him.

A very adventurous and capable American on a Caribbean island had built a small chocolate factory. He fixed things himself and made a nice profit. But he did not follow basic safety rules and electrocuted himself.

Good tools and good lighting are a must in every home, but tools can be dangerous. I know. I cut the tip off a finger rushing to do some woodwork with my favorite electric saw. Have flashlights everywhere. I use my shortened finger to remind me to be cautious. Don't rush. Whatever you do, take it easy.

Have your car inspected regularly. My neighbor thought to save money by skipping inspections, and one day she had a total brake failure. She was lucky and didn't get into an accident. Certainly, always wear a seat belt and keep a longer distance from the car in front of you than mandated. Let others cut in in front of you; don't teach them; teach yourself. If you take a defensive driving course on the Internet, you may learn something and get a discount on your car insurance.

Have smoke detectors everywhere and change the batteries regularly. I have a spare air tank handy at my bed side. In a fire, the poisonous fumes of plastics and smoke can kill you fast.

Don't live in a flood zone or high-risk forest fire zone. No government or insurance will protect you from your own bad choices. Make your home storm and weatherproof.

You may think of more hazards in house and garden, on the road, and in your hobbies. If you add them up, you will understand that chances for an accident are very high. In the worst case, you may hit your head and get a concussion with brain damage, just like what happened to my grandmother.

Preventing accidents costs you almost nothing. Having an accident is costly both to your health and finances. Please remember that accidents can be the leading cause of death in old age.

Before going to bed, Martha threw a towel down the stairs, planning to take it to the washing machine in the basement the next day. John, her husband, woke up at midnight and walked down to the kitchen to get a drink. He stepped on the towel, slipped, fell down the stairs, broke his neck, and was dead. Now Martha blames herself for having caused the accident.

While I am writing this, I read that Supreme Court Justice Ginsberg fell and broke some ribs for the second time. She is 85 but in excellent physical shape and works out every day.

I could have died in a fire on my boat. I tried to find and extinguish the source of heavy smoke, and I held a wet towel over my nose. Within a few breaths, I was dizzy and almost fainted.

Yea, yea, yea. You know all that. You most certainly know many more hazards in the house and garden, on the road, and in your hobbies.

Here are the three basic rules:

1. Think through every possible accident and emergency that can happen. How should you react? Help yourself first, so you can help others. Get help.
2. Take action now to avoid and prepare for accidents.
3. The first rule in an accident is: don't make it worse. Don't panic and don't rush. Take a deep breath and think for a few seconds. Those seconds can save a life.

On the other hand, if an accident happens, you will learn. For sure, you will be more careful about the rest of your life.

If, however, we consider aging another curable disease, then we might say the leading cause of death is not heart disease but aging.

4. Staying Fit Mentally and Physically

When you are over 80 or 90, what's the purpose of jogging and exercising in the gym? Sure, not being overweight helps prevent heart disease. But why fitness?

In the last chapter, we talked about preventing accidents, and being fit certainly helps.

But will fitness help you enjoy your last 20 years?

For millions of years, the fittest survived, and humans evolved by being fit. Fitness meant your capability to perform certain survival tasks. That meant climbing trees, picking fruit, catching prey, walking long distances, defending oneself, and adapting to harsh environments. Today, only a few jobs or professions require fitness for work. In the police, you need to run fast, lift people, or wrestle. As a bus driver, you may have to help passengers in an emergency.

Our lifestyle has changed dramatically as we evolved over millions of years. We were born to be fit. Just watch 2-year-olds; how they run, jump, swing their arms, preparing for the way humans lived millions of years ago. But now, most of us just need to be fit enough to push a button or say the words "Light on." We sit motionless in a car or airplane for hours. We sit in front of computers. We hardly ever climb stairs or lift heavy loads. And if we occasionally exercise, we get leg cramps or back pain.

Will this lifestyle lead to the extinction of the human species? Are we on the way to becoming sick and fragile, kept happy by drugs and passive entertainment? Are we losing interest in reproduction? All affluent societies are showing these trends.

But let us not get too far afield. The purpose of this book is not to extend the life of the species nor solve all of society's political and economic problems. All we want is to live, healthy and happy, for the last quintile of our life.

Exercise does not have to be strenuous. Easy walking, swimming, simple gymnastics, and easy sports can benefit you just as much as extreme gymnastics or performance sports. Regular exercise under the direction of a certified fitness trainer can prevent back pain, osteoporosis, joint problems, and cardiovascular problems. Therefore, staying fit is one key to a happy and healthy old age.

However, the most underrated effect of exercise is mental fitness.

At age 85, over 20 percent of people have some degree of dementia. Physical and mental exercise can delay or possibly prevent dementia such as Alzheimer's and other brain disorders, including stroke. The connection between exercise, both physical and mental, with just about every function or malfunction in your body is explained in Part II of this book. Although the causes of many neurological disorders are not completely understood, it is well known that smoking, obesity, high cholesterol, poorly controlled diabetes, and untreated high blood pressure increase the incidence of such diseases.

Even if you already suffer from a neurological disease, you will be able to deal with it much better if you are fit.

How fit do you have to be? To understand fitness in the context of a happy and healthy life after 80, we might look at the opposite. What is unfitness? You surely know many examples of physical and mental unfitness: your muscles feel tired, you should take a walk, but you find excuses. You rise out of a chair with some difficulty, walk upstairs slowly and breathing hard. You forget where you put things, forget names, and forget things you wanted to do, or don't remember your phone number. You listen to the news, but don't follow exactly what is being said. You have pains and aches in your back, your hip, and your shoulders. Arthritis inhibits your movements. Your weight is too high.

These are manifestations of unhealthy aging. You may tolerate them for a while. However, these symptoms will become more severe with time. The real aging has occurred during the 20 years before these symptoms become visible. It has occurred due to a lack of exercise, eating too much junk food, sleep deprivation, and the other things I talk about.

Dynamic fitness reduces and delays the symptoms of aging. Above all, it puts you in a positive state of mind. You walk faster and look forward to your daily exercise although you are tired. You get out of bed and start an active, enjoyable day. In summary, you feel better, are in command of your life, and are more likely to stay healthy.

How to become and remain fit? What does it take to be fit? For substantial health benefits, adults should participate in aerobic physical activity of moderate intensity for at least 150 minutes a week, or 75 minutes a week of vigorous intensity. Aerobic activity should be performed in episodes of at least ten minutes, and preferably, it should be spread throughout the week.

My daughter, who is a fitness trainer, reports that most clients initially want to lose weight. That's primarily about appearance and status. Anything wrong with that? Certainly not. But it wears off. Two months after the New-Year's resolution, only half the people participate. Unfortunately, it takes three months to start making exercise a habit.

Going to a gym is in fashion. To make a profit, the gym has to make exercise fun. They also have to guide and motivate you.

Those who stick with it experience something that we all love: feeling good. Instead of using drugs, your body produces its own feel-good chemicals, and you get addicted to exercise.

Besides physical fitness, there is brain fitness. The brain controls all the physical and chemical functions in your body. So, mental fitness is the key for overall fitness. Part II of this book explains the biological details of an aging brain. Again, mental fitness is not a static condition, such as intelligence. It varies and is the product of dynamic activity. It requires the stimulation of brain cells and their connections. Keeping the brain fit is not just a matter of blood circulation. It derives from the chemical and electrical activity of billions of neurons. It requires brain activity. We will get into all of that later.

The hardest part of exercise, physical or mental, is getting started. Motivating yourself is essential, particularly in the beginning and also when exercise becomes strenuous or boring or conflicts with other activities.

A very effective motivation for exercise is social: Join with friends, play with your grandchildren, look for a hiking group, or run with your dog. There are groups of birdwatchers, kayakers, and bocce players. Others are looking to go to lectures, concerts, and plays.

Look for anything that makes physical and mental exercise enjoyable. What is the most beautiful environment that you can experience by boat or bike, walking, jogging, or on horseback, swimming or snorkeling, in mountains, parks or on rivers, beaches, and lakes? Try combining travel with exercise. The same applies to mental activity. It is great to learn history as part of a group trip to a place where it happened.

Instead of jogging, I recommend "wogging," walking to the next telephone pole and then jogging to the next as slow as possible. Start with the absolute minimum effort, distance, and time. Never force yourself, never make exercise a punishment. Rest when you don't feel like working out. Fundamentally, your body wants exercise alternating with rest.

You can also exercise in bed or on a soft foam mat or in comfortably warm water. Wear comfortable clothing and shoes.

The next hurdle is staying with it. Avoid bad experiences. When you don't feel up to it, skip a day.

Again, work on motivation. Enjoy the fresh air, the scenery, or wear your earplugs and listen to your favorite tunes... Set yourself short-term and long-term achievable goals.

And work on your mental fitness. If you relax for four weeks doing nothing but laying on the sun deck of a cruise ship, your brain will get slow and dull. You need mental stimulation. Read a book, play tough games, learn something, take a course, discuss hot issues. Go back to school. Teach and coach. Your brain needs diversity.

5. You are what you eat

There are two primary biological purposes for eating and drinking: first, to supply energy to the body for daily work; and second, to supply building materials for the continuous growth of the billions of cells which comprise our tissues and organs.

Our metabolism has developed over millions of years. You can tell by our teeth that we were plant eaters. We climbed down from treetops and explored the savannah to harvest grain, roots, and berries. We also started hunting and followed the migrating herds of animals. Meat supplies a lot of energy, but berries, fruits, and vegetables provided the minerals and vitamins that we also need.

For millions of years, people never thought about health food. We ate what gave us energy and was not poisonous. That all changed with agriculture. Humans multiplied quickly because of the abundance of grain supplemented with meat from domesticated animals. That started humans down the path to an unhealthy diet. For 10,000 years, people ate what we now call "junk food" and paid with their health.

We have known for some time about the importance of a balanced diet as well as the danger of too much cholesterol, saturated fat, salt, and sugar. Nonetheless, much of what we eat is utter junk like soft drinks, fries, donuts, hot dogs, ice cream, and brain poisons like alcohol. Much of what you read about nutrition is advertising and just plain wrong. For example, most of the vitamins that people purchase are not necessary and simply go out with the next urination. Diet is determined more by convenience and advertising than anything else.

The most common justification for junk food is "it tastes good." Taste, however, is something that is strongly influenced by culture, including advertising. It is a vicious cycle: Our taste is a result of junk food and results in our eating more junk food.

Likewise, smoking cigarettes is extremely unhealthy. It results in heart disease, lung disease, and a variety of cancers. The packaging contains these warnings, yet many people smoke. Now, the companies who brought us this decidedly unhealthy practice are switching over to e-cigarettes or vaping. You can fulfill your nicotine addiction from a device instead of a cigarette. Is it safe? Of course not.

a) You are a Chemical Factory: Metabolism

Metabolism is what our body does with food. After food intake and digestive breakdown, the usable absorbed contents get widely distributed by the blood stream to all the cells of the body. A "food kitchen" inside each cell converts the food to energy for the cell and thereby powers all our muscles, nerves, and organs. It, too, is a great miracle of the evolution of life. There are trillions of chemical reactions taking place at any time. Our body is a huge chemical factory fed by carbohydrates, fats, proteins, water, oxygen, minerals, and vitamins.

Certain cells specialize in producing not energy but building materials for new cells. The blueprint for what to build is in the DNA of every cell. Each specialized cell knows what to produce for what purpose. Unlike industrial factories, there are no mechanical motors or pumps. All production of energy, enzymes, hormones, tissues, bones, muscles, nerves, and hundreds of glands and organs is highly dependent on a flawless interdependent system of osmosis and other mechanisms of transport within and through cell walls.

To give more excitement to the process, we have billions of little helpers in our body, namely bacteria. Both within our digestive tract and on the surface of our skin, we support many varieties of bacteria that feed on and live inside our body. Some of these friendly residents kick out disease-causing bacteria which have come to make trouble.

b) Naked on the Scale

You know what you eat and drink has great impact on your fitness and your health. That's not new. I won't bore you with things you already know like eating fewer calories and more vegetables.

Eating makes you feel good. Going out and socializing is enjoyable, especially when accompanied by some "street food." You have a craving for sweets and ice cream. You love baking with high-fat butter. A cold beer, a delicate cocktail, a glass of wine with good company; all that makes life worthwhile... and short.

Being hungry does not feel good. Being a party pooper by not drinking makes you an outcast. Watching others order a desert hurts. Meals without salt and fat just don't taste as good.

You are in a terrible dilemma. Right? Wrong! You are smart, and you have learned to motivate yourself for fitness and an enjoyable, healthy lifestyle. So, here is your plan:

Start with knowing the physical facts.

Step on a scale every morning, naked, after the toilet and before breakfast. Keep a fitness diary and record your meals and weight. You will quickly learn what adds weight and what does not. Surprise: often, very enjoyable meals don't add weight. Hamburgers and pizza add weight. Fatty sashimi or two big bowls of vegetable soup do not. If you want to lose weight, drink water before and with meals, eat apples, and eat just a little less. One of my friends says, "The way to ruin a good meal is to overeat!"

Eating is a habit, and taste is a learned attitude. If you need to feel stuffed to relax from stress, you have a problem. Meditate to change your self-image. You can program yourself for likes and dislikes.

The Northern European habit of eating a solid lunch and a very light and early supper makes you sleep well and digest better.

There is one proven secret for a longer life, at least in mice and rats. I have talked to people swearing by it. Religions practice it. And we can observe it in the whole animal world: fasting occasionally.

Getting used to ending a great meal by not stuffing everything in your tummy that mother has cooked. She will say: "Don't you like my food?" My mother pressured me into eating all that's on the plate with desert. She even forecasted good weather if I ate up. However, we might assume that during our evolution being hungry once in a while was probably more normal than routinely overeating.

c) You Are Still In The Stone Age

It is not necessary to study nutrition in order to eat right. Just remember that our digestive system and metabolism developed over millions of years. Eat a balanced diet like hunters and gatherers in the Stone Age and avoid the processed food of our industrial age.

A mix of berries, nuts, grain, greens, and some proteins from chicken or fish will be perfect.

People started processing healthy natural food into unhealthy processed food a long time ago. It started with fermenting fruit juice into alcohol and using smoke as a meat preserver. Additional preservation methods became necessary for mass distribution in the industrial age. Hardening margarine and cooking oils to prevent them from oxidizing was probably the worst thing, and it is still practiced. Hydrogenated fats clog our arteries and may stiffen cell membranes. Chemicals to avoid oxidization and infestation are used widely in industrial farming. Flavor and color additives are synthetically produced without regard for their impact on the complex chemical reactions in our body.

When you are 80 and plan to go to 100, and you have put on weight from eating pancakes, burgers, steaks, and French fries, it is not too late. If you start to eat mostly cholesterol-free foods and stick to polyunsaturated oils and fats, vegetables, fruits, and light, protein-rich meals, you will see a difference in your body within four to six weeks. Your skin will be smoother. You will lose weight, your cholesterol will come down, and if combined with regular exercise and plenty of water, you will be a different person within a year.

It may not be possible to reverse clogged arteries, but you can stabilize and, over the next ten years, even improve the condition, feel better, and decrease the likelihood of strokes and heart attacks.

Your most important meal is breakfast. Here is what I recommend: a variety of different fruits in a cup of nonfat yoghurt with a tablespoon of fish oil and half a teaspoon of cinnamon, a blood thinner. There is fish oil with lemon flavor in case you don't like the fishy taste.

The next most important meal is lunch. It should include some vegetables, for example a tomato, a stick of celery, green pepper, broccoli, and a carrot or a bowl of mixed salad. You may chop vegetables and spread it on a full-grain slice of bread with cream cheese.

In-between snacks should include some slices of apple. Apple gelatin lubricates the intestines. Afternoon tea and a slice of bread with jam is a habit invented by farmers to reduce the hunger of the working people before dinner. It may work for you too.

Dinner should be very light and easily digestible. Things like minestrone soup, a chicken salad sandwich, a sandwich with natural cheese, or a bowl of oatmeal. Reduce any fatty foods, particularly fried or roasted foods. Fried and roasted aromatic oils and fats can create free radicals, which are cancer-promoting substances. More about the causes of cancer later.

Among beverages, the best one is water. Drink at least a cup or two in the morning. Fruit juices can be added but not overdone. Coffee and tea are OK, but non-roasted ingredients should be preferred. Green tea is better than coffee. If you drink alcohol, a brain poison, you may prefer a glass of red wine a day which may have some antioxidants that are good for your heart (but probably not enough to make a difference). Avoid any high-calorie drinks like soft drinks.

In summary, the key to healthy nutrition is eating lots of organic fruits and vegetables supplemented with carbs from whole grain bread and proteins from fish, chicken, and low-fat dairy products. It is great when you get used to enjoying a healthy, tasty variety of foods and beverages.

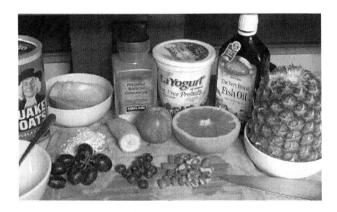

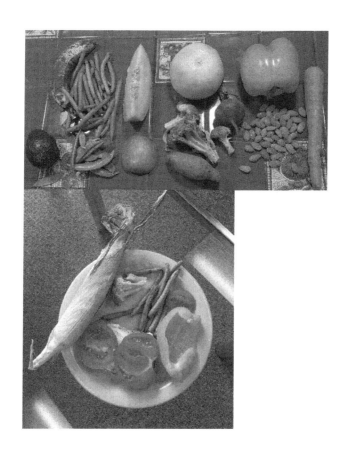

6. Health

What is health?

a) Absence of Illness?

There are many different definitions of good health. Most people will say, "If I feel well and have no pain, I am healthy."

But look at the weekend crowd in any restaurant. You see a lot of overweight 60-year-olds that are in good spirits. Are they healthy?

Yes, certainly, they might say. Their last physical showed a slightly high cholesterol, a bit of extra weight, but essentially good health.

Ten years later, the doctor prescribes Lipitor, exercise, and a healthier diet. The patient complies, and ten years later, well, you guessed it, a triple-bypass coronary operation.

So, at age 60, was that health? Or was it a lifestyle that ultimately leads to poor health?

I am alluding to the usual definition of health as the absence of illness or disease.

A better definition is: "**Health** is a state of complete physical, mental, and social well-being and not merely the absence of disease or infirmity."

That includes the lifestyle and mental determination to live a healthy life.

1. Healthy nutrition.
2. Regular physical activity
3. Regular medical checkups
4. Avoiding accidents

We have abandoned the lifestyle of millions of years where we were living in small communities while walking and working physically in fresh air. When hungry and tired, people gathered a variety of food. We still have the same body and metabolism, but we are sitting in front of a computer, in a car, or in front of a TV set overeating processed food. To make it worse, we are breathing exhaust-enriched air.

We can't go back and live like we are in the Stone Age, but we can be informed, read, Google, or ask a doctor. We have knowledge about our personal and environmental risk factors including the quality of air, water, food, and even noise. Then there is the issue of decreasing risk and avoiding accidents which I've already gone into in some detail. But there is another factor in increasing the odds for staying healthy, the most important one: determination and commitment to health. We must believe that it matters to decrease risk factors. We must believe that it matters to re-structure our environment, relationships, jobs, residence, and habits to prolong health and happiness.

b) Gamble With Your Life – And Win

Before we proceed to get further into how to stay healthy, we need to discuss something that none of us like to think about. What we are constantly discussing in this book is probability, a matter of odds. For example, eating healthy food and doing regular exercise will make it more likely that you will stay healthy and live longer than those who eat junk food and don't exercise. But it is not a sure thing! You are increasing your odds significantly, but there is always the possibility that the low frequency event will occur. Even when you cross the street obeying the traffic light and look both ways, there is the possibility for a low frequency event to occur. A speeding car may come out of a side street or driveway and mow you down. It's not your fault, and you made the right call to cross, but you end up severely injured or dead.

So, too, with illness. Some illnesses strike without warning, even in people who follow all the rules for healthy living. Breast cancer can affect women in their 30s before mammography is even suggested. A person may have a brain bleed from an unknown weakness in a cerebral artery. An incidental infection with a resistant bacterium can kill in a matter of days even with the best available medical care. No one is immune from bad luck. Doing everything right will not always work.

On the other hand, someone who smokes two packs of cigarettes per day may never get lung cancer, emphysema, or heart disease. They have lucked out. They bet a long shot and won.

The important thing to take from the phenomena of odds and luck is that we should not blame the victim of illness or accident for their trouble. Even more importantly, when we ourselves fall sick or are injured, it is likely we did nothing wrong. We were just unlucky. We may suffer from an illness that could not be prevented or an accident that could not be anticipated.

It is also true that had we known in advance that the illness was likely, we might have done something different. But that is not the point. It is bad enough to be the victim. Don't also blame yourself for what is not under your control.

Instead, focus on recovery and coping. We will address that topic in part II of the book in a well-referenced consideration of resilience.

In conclusion, life is a gamble, a matter of probabilities. Nothing is for sure, but the probabilities are in your hand, not by small margins. Smoking or not smoking, wearing a seatbelt or not, eating junk food or healthy food, exercising or not, getting health checkups or not, and many other choices increase the odds by huge margins.

c) The Living Cell

So here, finally, is the biological definition of health: "*Health* is the level of functional and metabolic efficiency of a living organism." That applies to every living being, even plants.

Fundamentally, life is not the body, but the cell, which is the building block of all life. The cell combines and controls all life functions— the design and construction of a tree or a flea, bacteria, a flower, an embryo, or a whole human person.

A single cell is a very complex factory with computer-like programs, chemical production, sensors, and transmitters of chemical and electrical signals. The cell communicates with trillions of other cells by electrical and chemical signals. Everything we eat, breathe, or feel influences this complex mechanism that is the essence of life.

Let's look at the evolution of the living cell.

When our planet cooled down, about 4.2 billion years ago, steam became water. Volcanoes threw up ashes and gases making for a smelly, boiling brew of sludge in which thousands of large molecules were formed from hydrogen, nitrogen, oxygen, carbon, cyanide (a carbon atom triple bonded to a nitrogen atom), and more.

Some molecules grew and grew, broke apart, combined with others, split again, and grew again. And by chance, one among trillions of such reactions became a molecule that would persistently fetch other molecules (DNA). The organizing principle was the shape, design, and size of the molecule which united with other molecules into more complex forms called polymers. These membranous droplets formed protocells, and these are the first cells.

These first cells likely included a minimal fatty membrane and initially just one gene that conferred some advantage to the cell. Later on, many of these very simple cells evolved by adding more genes. This type of simple cell persists until today. They are called prokaryotes. In fact, bacteria are prokaryotes. They have hundreds or even thousands of genes, but still multiply by simple division. Each daughter cell is exactly like the mother cell with the same DNA. Multiplication can be quick, with some bacteria in favorable environments doubling in number within 20 minutes. Like the rest of anything living, prokaryotes, and even simpler forms of life like viruses which cannot multiply on their own but need host cells to procreate, utilize the magic molecule for reproduction (i.e. DNA).

However, still another miracle occurred. One day, a primitive prokaryote ingested another, even smaller prokaryote which stayed alive inside the larger cell. This combination produced a much more complex and capable cell called a eukaryote. Eukaryotic cells have a nucleus (the old ingested cell) where most of the eukaryote cell's DNA resides. These more complex cells are the building blocks for all multi-cellular forms of life, both plant and animal, and even us!

Up to this day, all cells in our body change, get attacked by other cells and organisms, develop defense mechanisms, and fight for survival.

The cells in our body have developed quite a range of survival tactics. Not that they all stay alive and healthy all the time. Quite to the contrary, they split, multiply, and die. They are attacked by bacteria, viruses, and environmental factors. A mutation, an accidental mistake in coding DNA, may occur, and a faulty cell may still try to grow and reproduce. That might result in a cancer. But there is a police force, comprised of various types of white blood cells and immunoglobulins, which is on guard. It's a little like cops and robbers, and any little edge, such as good nutrition, exercise, sleep, etc., might determine the outcome.

Many cells produce enzymes, hormones, and all kinds of chemicals. In fact, a living being can be seen as a chemical factory. These chemicals control all life functions.

So, now the definition of health is not a static condition but an ever-lasting fight for survival of cells, of death and re-creation. It is an ongoing process. If that process works continuously well, it is health.

If it does not, we will see negative symptoms sooner or later, which we call illness. An illness is some kind of failure at the cellular level. Major causes are:

- Genetic, pre-programmed deficiencies in DNA replication that go along with increasing age. The overall plan seems to be to keep the species alive, not necessarily the individual.
- A mutated or inherited faulty DNA
- External interference, infections

- Chemical interference, bad nutrition, polluted air

Deficiencies often exist long before the whole machinery gives us trouble. For example, if our lifestyle weakens our immune system, we might not see any illness for years. But then, when we suffer diseases, the treatment often becomes complicated. We take several different medications, and each one has side effects. During our last quintile we become a great customer of the pharmaceutical industry. Do we have an alternative?

There is also a jungle of alternative treatments such as natural healing methods that people have used for thousands of years.

There is one healer that we know: built-in defense mechanisms. We have an incredible ability to heal. A cut in the skin attracts multiple enzymes that cause or promote pain, blood coagulation, white blood cells, healing, and nutrition for skin cells and more.

There are ways to activate our built-in healing system: Our mental condition, our lifestyle, and nutrition. Chicken soup promotes mucus and thereby may help recovery from the common cold.

But can we trust our natural healing system? Probably not; it also begins to deteriorate with age, especially if we have sinned against it for too long. And there is one built-in self-healing condition that we don't like: At some point our body may simply give up.

When does it no longer make sense to repair an old car? Unfortunately, many people want to stay alive at all costs even when in pain and with little likelihood of a future pleasant life. Our laws and current medical practice go along with such requests, and doctors are trained to keep patients alive. It often may not make sense.

Twenty-Five percent of Medicare's annual spending is used by the five percent of patients during the last 12 months of their lives. The trend is towards a very expensive prolongation of our life span with surgery, pills, transplants, DNA and stem cell manipulation, and other treatments still to be invented. Quality of life during that end stage may or may not be problematic for ourselves and loved ones.

Too little attention is given to other priorities, such as avoiding suffering, remaining mentally aware, spending time with friends and family, and not imposing burdens on others.

An alternative is palliative care. That involves visits from palliative care specialists, residential stays, and drugs and equipment that relieve suffering. Sometimes palliative care specialists work alongside the active treatment team, reminding all that patient comfort needs to be balanced against life extension.

d) Health Care

The annual physical is a start. Future monitoring will include complete monitoring of all types of cells, metabolism, organs, muscles, and even brain circuits. But we are getting ahead of ourselves. Let us return to the present.

Modern medicine has developed a whole range of diagnostic tools including CAT scans, MRIs, and even genome analysis of cancer cells. In addition to surgery and well-known medications like antibiotics and synthetic hormones (e.g. insulin and thyroxin), antidepressants and other psychiatric drugs have saved many lives and emptied out most mental hospitals. Medicines to control blood pressure, blood sugar, cholesterol, and blood clots in vulnerable people are just a few examples of great preventative advancements. Early detection of breast cancer with mammography and regular colonoscopies to find colon polyps before they grow into cancers have saved many lives. These are just examples. New procedures like gene therapy, immunotherapy, and stem cell transplants are supplementing or replacing older forms of cancer treatment. If you are well, do the things we recommend in this book. If you get sick, please go to the doctor. In fact, older people should, at the very least, go for an annual physical exam and have their medications reviewed.

You probably have had a doctor for a long time who knows you and cares about you. If you don't, or if you want to change, it is not easy to evaluate doctors. I found that ratings by patients mean nothing. Those ratings refer to friendliness but do not address professional competence. I don't have the perfect answer, but I believe in four criteria for a good doctor:

1. Teaching requires staying up to date, so all things considered it might be best to search for a doctor who is part of an academic medical system. That affiliation also may provide quick access to appropriate specialty care as needed.
2. You have to strike it right in relating to the doctor. Have a conversation. Discover mutual interests and friends. I

worry that some doctors write off health problems of old people as just a result of old age.
3. If you detect anything like a lack of interest or lack of professionalism, change immediately and look for another doctor. Never hesitate to get a second opinion.
4. Look for very thorough analysis and diagnostics by the doctor and the staff.

If your health has deteriorated, you might take along a relative or close friend to help you remember what the doctor said. It also provides another opinion about the doctor.

7. Care and Nursing homes

a) Search and Plan Well

Some day you may want help with your daily activities. Trading your familiar home for a new environment, albeit one with readily available physical assistance, meals, housekeeping, perhaps more social contacts, and on-site professional care is not a simple decision. If you want to compare the pros and cons of retirement communities, assisted living, and nursing homes with help or care at your home, you can get advice from Medicare, your doctor, township counselors, or from books. Browsing the internet, courses, and lectures will also provide information. Even more useful is visiting family and friends already experiencing care.

This website is quite useful:

https://www.medicare.gov/NursingHomeCompare

Since what is at stake is so important, you should start your information gathering years before you need the service. If necessary, family and friends can help you with the research.

Do not fall victim to salespeople and organizations which promise a lot. Their main goal may be extracting as much money from you as possible.

There are great differences in cost, performance, security, options, and the subsequent possibility for comfort and enjoyment.

b) Good Company

Nothing will make you happier than being surrounded with nice people, including friendly staff, in whatever help facility or arrangement you select. Staying or moving close to family and friends should also be a priority.

Most people prefer to live at home but owning a house may require more work and cost than moving to a condo or even a senior-living community with services. Other residents with similar interests can be a real bonus as one gradually loses old friends over time.

Living in a retirement community may cost less than your own home since the space is smaller, and you have no backyard or garden. Instead, there may be a park-like environment and community facilities. Some facilities are located in high-rise buildings; others are single-family villas. These are not nursing homes with care services, but some have a nursing office, and you are free to hire outside help.

If you have a spouse or partner, particularly if one of you can still drive safely, you can live quite economically.

Many retirement communities offer an ideal climate. Some locations in wooded areas, near lakes, or at higher altitudes may be healthy, enjoyable, and much less expensive than others near popular beaches or famous resort areas. However, many retirees miss their grandchildren or develop serious health problems. After a few years, they re-locate again to be closer to family. Another issue is how well do you adapt to new environments. Visit the place and look at the design, the view, surroundings, air, and climate---both summer and winter. Talk to residents, stay for breakfast, lunch, and dinner. Look at the programs for fitness, events, entertainment, studies, and courses. Check out the health care resources, living facilities, options for dining, and personal care. A healthy and pleasant climate and places with leisure activities like swimming, hiking, and other outdoor activities may help keep you healthy or mitigate the problems you already have. But there is also the possibility that you will get sick or an existing problem will worsen. Are there arrangements for higher levels of care like a nursing home?

Do this before you consider cost. Find out what the best of the best offer. The more you see, the better will be your decision.

c) The Cost of Care

The greatest cost factor is the state of your health. Do you only need help with your household duties, or do you need around-the-clock intensive personal care, like showering, toileting, getting out of bed or a chair, walking, taking medications, and eating? Find out the cost for each type of care.

Many continuing care facilities will formally assess your health, particularly if they offer to guarantee your lifelong care after entrance. Even more important than your physical state, they will assess your mental state, as the cost of dementia care is very high, and the condition can go on for many years.

If there is evidence that health is becoming compromised, either from a physical or mental perspective, it may be wise to consider an early move to a place that offers a variety of care options at a fixed price. That consideration is less important if one has already arranged for insurance to cover the possible need for nursing home, assisted living, or memory care facilities.

L. S. from Philadelphia was age 78, divorced, had two pensions and social security. He had refinanced his old house and spent the mortgage money and his savings on supporting his daughter and granddaughter. His health was relatively good, considering he had been a heavy smoker most of his life. He was playing golf and baseball until age 64, but then became very weak, had trouble walking stairs, did not see well, and felt he could not drive anymore. His daughter helped him find a nursing home nearby that would accept his income and charge the rest to Medicaid. He had to share a room with another person, but he liked the company. He didn't like the food, but his daughter visited him and invited him over for dinner occasionally. He died of heart failure five years later.

Not every nursing home accepts patients without payment. But since Americans age 65 to 74 have a median retirement savings of $125,000 with only social security income, many patients come in on a self-pay basis, but will depend on Medicaid sooner or later. About 65 percent of nursing home residents are supported primarily by Medicaid.

The background for this phenomenon is that federal law requires all states to provide nursing facilities for Medicaid recipients. States must also pay for Medicaid-eligible home health care services for recipients who would otherwise qualify for nursing home care. There are strict financial audits before certifying a patient as eligible for Medicaid. In addition, there is rule-based medical necessity certification required before Medicaid pays for nursing home care. Assuming your house is worth $100,000, your retirement funds worth $50,000, and your monthly social security income $1,500, you will most likely not be able to pay for a nursing home and will not qualify for Medicaid. You will have to find a nursing home that accepts your assets and savings as down payment for its fees. Only after your money and assets are completely used up will the costs shift over to Medicaid.

G.F. from New Jersey was in great health at age 90. She had a bad car accident, which was her fault. She felt that it was time to move to a facility with independent and assisted living options as well as a skilled nursing home on site. She felt that she could have managed at home with some outside assistance, but that might not last very long.

She sold her house for $155,000. She had savings from her late husband of $450,000 and social security income. She visited several facilities and decided on one in her neighborhood, next to a large mall and close to her friends. She paid down $90,000 and rented a small apartment with three meals but without assistance for $2,300 a month. She likes the company, participates in daily gymnastics, plays cards, and uses the shuttle bus for shopping while her car stays mostly in the parking lot. She complains about the food getting worse and is afraid of the financials down the road. The home must accommodate her for her life, even if her money runs out. But as of now, at age 93, she can cover her expenses. The home would provide daytime assistance for $20 an hour, but she was able to hire outside help twice a week for four hours for $15 an hour.

S.K. from New Jersey was 88, a bit overweight, with his right arm paralyzed. A retired engineer, he had a decent retirement account from his former employer, plus social security. His daughter living nearby tried to get him into a nursing home, but he wanted to stay at home. He needed help at home and for shopping and hired a woman from the neighborhood for $15 an hour, 5 days a week, 4 hours a day, and a former nurse, also from the neighborhood for $28 an hour, 4 hours every Saturday, who would check his medication and prescriptions and give him a good wash-down and a massage. His daily helper also drove him to the beach occasionally. In return, he paid her for her hotel room when they stayed overnight. His wife had passed away ten years ago. Nonetheless, he enjoyed living in his familiar old neighborhood.

His retirement fund withdrawals and social security could well cover his home insurance, taxes, maintenance, and landscaping of $24,000 a year, and his help of $21,000 a year. He was not much concerned with his health, and he died of heart failure at age 89.

R.S. of New Jersey was 102 years old, and his spouse, I.S., was 79 years old. The two had savings of $3.6 million from the sale of R's former company, which was invested in bonds and stocks, allowing a withdrawal of $70,000 a year without reducing the balance. In addition, they received $2,300 a month of social security, and she drove a school bus for the township, which covered the health insurance of the couple. At age 99, he suffered a mild stroke but was still able to do his daily walk around the block. He had never been active in sports except leisurely golf, while she swam a mile every day and rode her bike on weekends. Both were in great health, but at age 100, he fell at home and had another stroke. This time, his memory was severely damaged, and he needed daytime assistance if his wife was out of the house. He hated the daytime assistant. Although he wanted to stay in their beautiful home, his wife looked around for the best continuing care community facility in the area. They paid down $500,000 and rented a three-room apartment with three meals a day for $6,000 a month. The facility offered daytime assistance for $25 an hour but they hired outside help 4 hours on weekdays for $15 an hour. So far, it has worked out well. He is 103 and 6 months and still in relatively good health but can only walk with assistance or a walker.

My last example is a bit more serious. E.P., now 81, had been in good health. She had a small business with one employee. At age 78, she suddenly could not remember simple things, like amounts of money. Her loss of memory quickly progressed, and she was diagnosed with Alzheimer's. Her daughter researched memory care units in nursing homes. By the time she arrived at the unit, six months later, she had no memory about her business and could not even remember her children.

Presently, three years later, she is still in good health except for her loss of memory. She can move around well, eat, drink, but needs 24-hour assistance, for which the home offers several price categories.

The down payment was $120,000, and the monthly cost for a one-bedroom, one-living-room apartment with all meals and assistance is $8,800 a month. Her assets should be sufficient for ten more years. She cannot be evicted, and Medicaid will pay for the cost once her money runs out. The quality of the home is excellent, although her daughter thinks the food is not the best and visits her often and takes her home for dinner.

If you do not qualify for Medicaid, you might consider staying in your own home, particularly if one spouse can help the other. That involves house management, arranging for help, shopping, and organizing medications and finances.

Visiting Angels charges $24 per hour for daytime care at home or $230 a day for live-in care, including personal care.

Another possibility is help from family. Historically, families took care of the elderly, who in turn helped around the household, baby sat, and shared their wisdom and experience with younger family members.

The family might choose to help with home expenses and repairs, as well as shopping and driving, especially to medical appointments.

Some families choose to invite a parent or other elderly relative into a spare bedroom; other families choose to build an addition onto their house. Handrails and ramps often are very helpful. A private entrance is a possibility.

Other couples choose to move to a low-cost country. That requires being comfortable living in a different culture and possibly learning a different language. I met a couple that sailed to the Dominican Republic and built a house in a beautiful shore area. All their costs including very inexpensive local help was less than their social security income. There are very affordable American retirement communities in several Central and South American countries. Medical care for serious illnesses can be a problem and may require flying to the U.S.

If you want to live in luxury at a total cost of living for a couple of under $2,000 per month including local health care, you

might consider investigating the following countries listed by International Living Magazine:
1. Nicaragua
2. Thailand
3. Costa Rica
4. Malaysia
5. Spain
6. Malta
7. Ecuador
8. Mexico
9. Portugal
10. Panama

These websites are a helpful start in your research:

https://internationalliving.com
https://longtermcare.acl.gov/pathfinder/65plus.html

Below are some national average costs for long-term care in the United States in 2016. Average costs for specific states are also available.

https://www.genworth.com/aging-and-you/finances/cost-of-care.html

This article by Medicare informs you about 11 alternatives to nursing homes:

https://www.medicare.gov/nursinghomecompare/Resources/Nursing-Home-Alternatives.html

8. Money

Work in retirement does not have to be for money. You could work for fun or volunteer for the benefit of organizations you value. Churches, hospitals, organizations for the needy, and local schools are all looking for volunteers. Friends and neighbors sometimes need help. Volunteer work may provide benefits other than cash. One great benefit of working is keeping your brain active.

If you have three million or more dollars in your retirement fund plus social security or a pension plan, you don't have a financial problem. If you have $200,000 or less and social security, if you run into serious infirmity, you will be eligible for a Medicaid-supported nursing home. But what if you are somewhere in between and need to earn money? What are your options?

The answer depends on when you start planning. At age 80, it's a bit late, although if you could generate some additional income, you might live more comfortably. Ideally, you should make plans no later than at age 45, when you still have an income. At that time, all you need is pencil and paper and the will to make a budget. If you make the right investment decisions, your nest egg will grow to a comfortable size by the time you reach age 80.

Consider also the possibility that by age 80, you might be richer than expected. You might still have a sizeable income of interest, pension, social security, and capital gains if you sell your real estate or other assets. Taxes are likely to grow, so I recommend putting your investments in a Roth plan, where you pay taxes earlier, compared to an IRA where you pay income taxes later upon withdrawal.

The most important investment rule is to diversify. Unless you are an experienced investor with enough resources to diversify on your own, mutual funds or exchange traded funds (ETFs) are likely the best way to go. Look for low management fees and no sales charge. There are investment funds for stocks and other investment funds for bonds; some investment funds are "balanced," in that they invest in both stocks and bonds. Check the long-term performance of any funds you plan to buy. Then sit back and relax. Check your funds' performance at least monthly, but not too frequently, as the daily fluctuations of the stock and bond markets mean little. The advice of brokers and investment advisers may or may not be useful. Of course, be especially careful of any gains they might accrue from selling you any particular fund. Friends are another peril. They always have "great investment ideas." Courses on investments of any kind are generally sponsored by someone who wants your money. Be skeptical and don't rely on one opinion. An unbiased source for financial information and education is the paper "Investor's Business Daily." Savings accounts at the bank currently earn next to nothing. Plan for an annual inflation of two to three percent and aim for a withdrawal of three to four percent annually without decreasing your assets. Don't pay interest on credit cards. Instead, obtain a bank loan at a lower rate of interest to pay off the credit card debt.

A great way to stay abreast of your investments is to form or join an "investor club." This is a group of friends, who meet weekly or bi-weekly and discuss their portfolios or even invest in a joint portfolio. You elect a target market and a stock. In a rotating order, one member researches a company, its owners, managers, its market, its competitors, and its history. This is an interesting social activity and can be quite lucrative.

Bonds and stocks often move in opposite directions, and many people use both to partially protect against the chance of a recession or alternatively a period of great inflation. In a recession, the stock portion of your portfolio will move down in value, but the bonds you own will be stable or tend to move up as interest rates fall.

On the other hand, stocks are a good hedge against inflation as they generally represent the value of the underlying businesses. Diversification is likely the best strategy, even though the stock market usually outperforms the bond market over a period of time.

Think twice about buying the highest yielding investments. They are likely the most risky. One type of low risk investment is an inflation-protected bond. However, the interest rate is likely relatively low.

Again, as we get older, the best advice is to diversify and avoid too much risk. We cannot afford to lose the money we need to live on. None of the above is meant to be investment advice.

The tougher question is how to generate income when you are old and nobody wants to hire you.

One simple solution is to work for yourself. Be an independent contractor and set up your own company. That can be a simple as watching homes for people on vacation.

Answer four questions:

1. How much do you need to earn? Make a budget and consider a few worst-case scenarios of unforeseen expenses.
2. How much do you really like to work?
3. What are your skills and favorite activities? Write down your strengths and weaknesses.
4. Search for opportunities that meet above criteria.

Let's make the following assumptions:
You expect to be five years away from needing senior care. You have budgeted all income and expenses, all assets, and have made a savings plan, but you need another $200,000.

You want to be flexible in your time and work a maximum of four hours a day, five days a week. Let's say 40 weeks a year. That would be an income of $1000 a week or $200 a day or $50 an hour.

Low-skill home services earn $15 an hour and up to $30 an hour with some skills. Part time jobs (e.g., trade shows, events, hotels etc.) pay $8 to 15 an hour.

Arts and crafts earn less than that. Online Internet work, although promising up to $200,000 a year, delivers even less on average.

The key to earning more is to find your own little monopoly. Where you are the best, have little competition, and can deal with customers that value your services.

Can you combine your skills, your connections, and some equipment or assets? Can you organize and let others work for you, while you do the selling?

Look around at your neighborhood, your friends, clubs, and former employers. A stockbroker, real estate agent, accountant, or attorney who could continue business with his contacts in retirement, usually does not need the income. How about a relationship with someone who trusts you and lets you service former clients? Building trusting relationships should be started as early as possible and continued throughout your life.

Your service may be more profitable if it includes equipment that you operate.

One type of equipment you may have is your house. I recently stayed at a home that I rented through Airbnb. The owner rented three rooms to up to five people and was sold out almost every day for a total income of $300 a night, $2100 a week.

A friend in Grenada does house and boat watching. She lives in one of the houses she services, including caring for pets while the owners travel. She charges $80 a day per home, but has no expenses, other than her own food.

Another friend takes care of five multi-million-dollar homes in Florida for owners that rarely visit. He contracts workers and landscapers and pays all local fees and taxes. His income is $5,000 a month.

I met a lady in Munich, Germany, who has a small garden house in the outskirts of town and takes care of 12 dogs. Not just a kennel, she walks dogs and trains some of them. She earns $900 a day.

A friend in a California town sells landscaping to companies. His clients are a bank chain, several hotels, and some corporate headquarters. He is just the contractor and directs the landscapers. He earns around $8000 a month.

My dad, at age 72, got tired of not working, and was hired as a furniture salesman in a department store. He knew how to dress and talk and approach people, but had little hope of making much money, working only on commission and being by far the oldest salesperson. But, surprise, many rich and older customers wanted no other salesperson than my dad, who discussed their lifestyle, their home style, and asked the right questions. Soon, he had the most sales, even though he only worked 3 days a week during evening hours.

A local friend of 78 is a school bus driver for a township. She makes only $15 an hour, 6 hours a day but gets a very generous benefits program including health insurance for her family.

Driving an Uber or Lyft car is easy work, totally flexible and does not require any more skills than owning a car and being a safe and polite driver. Income is said to be $1000 to $2000 a month.

A boating friend of mine, age 88, qualified for a captain's license years ago. He teaches a safe-boating course twice a week. He gets an average of 100 participants paying $20 each, totaling $4000 a week. Less expenses for the room and share of his sponsor, a boat dealer, he earns $2400 a week.

Some of the above examples require skills, some not. Every profitable activity requires trust, people skills, a clean well-groomed appearance, and some effort in searching.

Trial and error with different activities will likely be necessary before you find your niche.

A bit of selling experience is always helpful:

- Have some knowledge about the business you are getting in
- Know your customer.
- Don't talk too much, listen carefully and let your customer talk.
- Print a business card and a pamphlet of what you offer, including your credentials.
- Have some references.
- Don't talk price until your fish has bitten the bait
- Go for the best opportunity
- Never do business with bad people

Here are some ideas for supplementary income.

http://www.aarp.org/work/working-after-retirement/info-03-2011/more-great-part-time-jobs-for-retirees.html

http://www.huffingtonpost.com/2012/07/03/retirement-jobs-part-time_n_1637229.html?slideshow=true#gallery/235693/0

One way to pay for long-term care while you still have an income and pay income taxes is a Health Savings Account (HSA). If you're covered by an eligible high-deductible health plan in 2019, you can contribute up to $3,500 for an individual or $7,000 for a family to an HSA, reducing your taxable income by that amount. HSA money is tax-free when withdrawn, provided it goes to pay medical, dental, or long-term care expenses. You can invest and let your money grow for decades tax-free so long as you or a surviving spouse eventually use it for medical expenses. An HSA can even serve as a backup rainy-day fund should you suddenly need cash. You can take money out tax-free to reimburse yourself for any prior years' medical expenses paid from outside the account. Plus, once you turn 65, you can withdraw money for nonmedical use.

If you put $7,000 a year into an HSA starting at age 35, you would have over $1 million at age 75, assuming growth plus interest of six percent per year.

9.   Life in Retirement

Any leisure activity that involves good company is good for health. Such activities can be hiking, birdwatching, biking groups, yoga, gymnastics groups, and travel groups.

Pets also may be thought of as pleasant companions. Dogs are social animals just like humans.

In addition to simple conversations or sharing of hobbies and games, activities that help others are gratifying. This can be coaching, teaching, counseling, guiding of tourists, hosting, hospice services, or volunteering for church, club, or school. Cooking and feeding the many homeless is another possibility.

A great combination of mental exercise and social activity is attending classes. They can cover a huge variety of subjects and are usually free for seniors at a community college. My old friend Milton, between age 90 and 100, attended classes about *History of Religions, German Language, Book Discussions,* and several history classes. Another friend was a fan of archeology and joined several study journeys to the Middle East.

Social interaction is so important that it should rank highly when and if you choose to move to any kind of retirement arrangement.

10. Happiness

a) The Happiest Moments in My Life

Think about the happiest experiences of your life. Envision the most enjoyable moments of your life. Keep those memories alive like a magic diamond. Write them down here:

1.

2.

3.

You know, of course, that such joyous moments cannot be permanent. There is no such thing as eternal happiness.

Look in the mirror and ask: Am I happy? Now smile and ask again. And then, ask: Well, when I look at the last ten years, not counting little ups and downs, am I generally a happy person?

So, already, you have three different definitions of happiness. And there are more. In fact, happiness per se is complicated and there are many definitions.

b) The Myth of Happiness

While Beethoven calls joy a spark of the gods in his "Ode an die Freude" in his 9th Symphony, it is the devil in "Hoffman's Tales" that promises ultimate happiness.

Goethe's Faust had tried everything that science could offer to find happiness, but he could not find it. So, he made a pact with the devil, who would get his soul if he could provide total happiness. The devil supplied Faust with every imaginable pleasure on Earth but could not satisfy him. At last, Faust discovered that by building dams against ocean floods, he saved thousands of lives, and much to the dismay of the devil, his last words were that this was the moment of highest happiness that he wanted to last.

Zum Augenblicke dürft' ich sagen:
Verweile doch, du bist so schön!
Es kann die Spur von meinen Erdentagen
Nicht in Äonen untergehn.—
Im Vorgefühl von solchem hohen Glück
Genieß' ich jetzt den höchsten Augenblick.

Here is my free translation:

This work, my strongest strive,
I call the highlight of my life
but, lasting for eternity,
My life on Earth will go away.
Remain, enjoyable serenity
This moment I may ask to stay.

The American Constitution hints in a similar direction with "….in pursuit of happiness…," implying that happiness is a pursuit rather than the final achievement. The State of Pennsylvania kept the phrase in its welcoming sign: "Pennsylvania… In Pursuit of Happiness."

Certain religions associate happiness with the afterlife. Striving for eternal happiness in Heaven; in other words, the pursuit of happiness is happiness on Earth.

There are a variety of myths that create happiness in their pursuit, such as fighting and dying for your country or working hard to accumulate wealth and education for your offspring, even if you never achieve the objective yourself.

Can you imagine devoting your life to a goal, feeling happiness in every step of the struggle?

c) Feeling Happy

Most essential for the survival of any species is reproduction. Consequently, the sexual process is associated with powerful positive feelings:

Your first love, marriage, and a baby are all usually very gratifying.

Even passing exams, finding a job, obtaining a raise, winning an award, buying a house or a car may be seen as related to survival of the human species. Those things also enhance self-esteem and increase social status.

These motivations for survival of yourself and your family occur relatively early in life. Once you are over 80 and no longer in the reproductive stage of life, the greatest happiness may be to see one's offspring be successful. Grandchildren give us great joy when they thrive.

d) Status

We are social animals, meaning we live in interacting tribes, communities, and groups that accept us and protect us. Survival of the species depends on a functioning social life. Individuals benefit from society, and society benefits from its members. Mutual help in nutrition, reproduction, and defense are key. Society judges and positions us relative to our social value.

Status reflects our place in society. It is all very hierarchical. We strive to be valued, respected, and liked. It starts with being rewarded by our mother for eating well. Our parents teach us to be good and not to engage in bad behavior. Later on, we strive to be good students. We compete in sports and play, and our friends let us know if we are good or bad. Suddenly, we discover conflicts between what parents and teachers tell us and what our friends tell us. Then once we change our social environment by going off to school or a job, we are influenced by different standards for acceptance.

The military teaches nationalism and honor, companies reward loyalty and diligence. Colleges reward academic accomplishment and sporting prowess. Our family expects us to do well financially and raise a family. Some families also implant the thirst for wealth and power.

If we fail, we may become sad, frustrated, desperate, sick, or depressed. If we become lost, isolated, and lonely, it may lead to depression. As we age, the stakes may get higher; we are running out of time to achieve success.

Having reached high status should give us satisfaction, but the dynamics of group standards and the fragility of our position never let us rest. Success does not necessarily make us happy, because that moment is fleeting. Rather, it is progressing towards success that gives satisfaction. People are different; some are happy with the status quo; others need continuous, challenging advancement.

The pertinent question for us is what will make us happy as we approach old age? How will we earn rewards, respect, praise, and love when we are over 80?

I have asked that question of old folks, friends, social workers, teachers, doctors, psychologists, and terminally ill patients. Here is what I heard back:

1. Give love and respect. You will receive respect and affection in return.
2. Join groups of your interest. Define your skills. Try to contribute value with your abilities. Play, travel, meet, perform, lecture, sing, teach, and study. Discuss with others how to improve the world and how to better your life. Find new friends of all ages. If alone, find someone special.
3. Create something. It could be something without monetary value, perhaps something that makes you feel proud of yourself. Gardening, art, writing, and home design are all possibilities. Or combine your activity with income. Money follows interest. Count your profit. Once you find your niche, go about implementing it; don't waste time.
4. Once you find what to pursue, study up. Interview people. Find a job just to learn and spy. Form your own company. Have your grandchildren set up your website and teach you how to blog.
5. If you do not discover something grand, enjoy little things. Dream, read, travel. Attend lectures, music, and theater.
6. The most used and least effective tool for searching for happiness is buying things. Cosmetic surgery is a close second.

e) Self- Esteem

As powerful as status may be in searching for happiness, it pales in comparison with self-esteem. Confidence in one's own worth and abilities, faith in oneself, pride, dignity, and morale are all part of self-esteem.

Much as we want others to like and respect us, they are not us. We live inside our own heads. Whatever others may say about us, we know the truth, or at least think we know the truth. There is always a witness to what we were thinking, what was the motivation, even what we actually saw when calling the tennis ball out of bounds.

Indeed, esteem from others and high status often conflict with what the individual feels inside. The thought inside is much more important. For example, if one is complemented for giving a great lecture, but the ideas were taken from another without proper acknowledgement, was it really a great lecture?

When individuals suffer from clinical depression, difficulty with self-esteem is what is most important. The more others tell them they are really a good person with much to live for, i.e. family who love them, co-workers who value them, great past accomplishments and an unlimited future, the more the depression strengthens as the individual feels that the praise is undeserved. Whether or not the outside praise is accurate or inaccurate is not particularly important. Self-esteem or the lack of it is what counts.

The phenomenon of self-esteem accounts for the inevitable surprise when a "successful person" commits suicide. To all outward appearances, the person is doing well--- educated, financially secure, has a loving spouse and children, well-respected, etc. Why does that person feel so terribly that they choose to die? The answer is often not simple. However, each and every person who attempts suicide at that moment feels terrible about themselves; their self-esteem has crashed, and what other people think is unimportant.

The evidence for the importance of self-esteem is not limited to depressed individuals. Even in much less crucial areas such as performance in sports, most participants are more interested in how they played (as assessed by themselves) than the final outcome. Each of us know that the score is not necessarily indicative of what really happened. It may be that you played badly, but the opponent played even worse or any number of other possibilities.

f) The Chemistry of Happiness

Neuroscientists have discovered that certain chemicals in the brain are associated with feeling good or bad. They are predominantly neurotransmitters which facilitate communication across synapses in the specialized brain circuits associated with the perception of happiness. Some of the best known are:

- Adrenaline, which is the fight- or-flight hormone. It provides for energy in emergency situations.
- Endorphins are painkillers that allow you endure extreme effort despite pain and exhaustion.
- Serotonin has some antidepressant activity and also decreases anxiety.
- Dopamine is a reward hormone. Naturally produced, it makes you feel happy.
- Oxytocin is produced by sexual activity, childbirth, and caressing or hugging.

These naturally occurring substances are necessary for our survival. They even provide a natural high in certain circumstances, as when, after intense exercise, there is great relaxation and almost a "high." You can get addicted to the great feeling after a good workout, overcoming the memory of hard work and fatigue. That is called a positive addiction.

Certain drugs, unfortunately, mimic endorphins and other brain chemicals. For example, opiates, cocaine, and amphetamines can fool the brain into temporary happiness. Nicotine and alcohol are similar but less powerful. This artificially created happiness de-activates the natural mechanisms for achieving happiness or calm, even overriding hunger, sexual desire, or other natural pleasures. Eventually, nothing works to relieve the depressed and anxious mood except these drugs of abuse in ever-increasing amounts. For many people, this result is a chronic battle with addiction; for others, there is a loss of interest in anything else but getting the drug to temporarily feel better. The amount of drug required keeps escalating, often resulting in accidental overdose. Just as commonly, the addict gives up. Life is over for them, and they commit suicide.

Substances that are commonly considered less harmful can also seriously damage health. Overeating as means of dealing with frustration can kill over time. Feeling too tired to exercise after a day of sitting in front of a computer is also not good for health. Alcohol to relax from stress may catch up to you in the last quintile of life.

For millions of years, humans fought adversaries or ran away for survival. Gathering food, fishing, hunting, and competing for mating were natural activities leading to happiness. Today, working eight hours, having regular meals, watching TV, meeting mates at dances or hobbies may be less powerful emotional rewards. No wonder drugs, alcohol, video games, movies, and restaurants are such big industries, rivaling the medical industry which is trying to repair the problems. It is the industrialization of happiness. Could such pursuit of passive happiness result in the ultimate downfall of the human species?

Before we leave the topic of the chemistry of happiness, perhaps let's discuss alcohol. There is no doubt that sometimes alcohol can cheer us up, especially if we are already in a good mood and surrounded by friends and fun. On the other hand, alcohol can make one feel more depressed if one is already feeling down.

Alcohol also figures prominently in accidents, especially motor vehicle accidents. But everyone already knows that. What about things that are less well known?

According to a 2008 study[14] in the *Archives of Neurology*, heavy drinking over a long period of time shrinks brain volume. The study of 1,839 subjects from the Framingham Offspring Study found that people who had more than 14 drinks per week over a 20-year timeframe had 1.6 percent smaller brains (a measure of brain aging) than those who were non-drinkers. Overall, the association was slightly stronger in women than in men. Drinking moderately was not protective. The more alcohol consumed, the smaller the total brain volume.

Heavy drinking also may speed up memory loss in early old age, at least in men, according to a 2014 study[15] in the journal *Neurology*. Men in the study who had more than two and a half drinks a day experienced signs of cognitive decline up to six years earlier than those who did not drink, had quit drinking, or were light or moderate drinkers.

g) Future and Present Happiness

Is there a recipe for long-term happiness? May it require sacrifices in the present pursuit of happiness? Can I train myself to enjoy being hungry in order to lose weight? Can I resist alcohol when I need to calm down from anger and stress? Can I overcome tiredness with exercise instead of resting? These are important questions which require an honest answer. Try to meditate and talk to yourself or ask a counselor for help

The Bible talks about the forbidden fruit in Paradise and the identification of immediate pleasure with sin. The struggle between what is pleasurable for us in the short run, but destructive in the long run is obviously a very old story.

h) Happy and Unhappy People

I asked my friend Milton at his 103rd birthday, "Are you happy?" He hesitated. His mind is not always there, and I thought he had fallen asleep. Then he answered, "Am I satisfied with my life? I think there is too much emphasis on money. I enjoy discovering something new every day."

"What have you discovered recently?"

"This soup," he said. "I never had such a soup. That's new. I learned something."

I asked several people from different backgrounds a simple question, "Are you happy?" And I got two different answers from two different types of people:

Most answered by stating several reasons that make them unhappy, then saying if it were not for those problems, they would be happy.

The other type, answered, yes, they were essentially happy, and they would list a number of reasons why they are happy, admitting there were occasional problems.

I followed up by asking what specifically made them happy or unhappy. The surprising result is that both types mentioned the same experiences leading to happiness or unhappiness.

Both had worries of various kinds: financial, kids, and health. The happy ones still considered themselves happy.

Many of the reasons mentioned for unhappiness were related to complaints about others. The people who presented reasons for unhappiness are "would-be-happy" people. Many of their problems are not serious, but they get upset easily, even by minutia.

On the other hand, I have met people who live on a meager pension, can't travel, have health problems, delay house repairs, and are totally happy. What is the difference?

Satisfying relationships are mentioned by psychologists as key to happiness. Some researchers hypothesize a genetic basis for happiness or unhappiness a bit like my speculation that there are two different types of people, happy and unhappy people.

Another difference between happy and unhappy people may be mental balance, an inner peace with oneself. These people seem to have less conflicts, stress, and fear. They have self-esteem and trust themselves to solve any problems that come their way.

It seems to me that people who live in peace and harmony with themselves and others have an understanding of life and themselves. They have a life philosophy or a religion; many practice meditation or yoga. In talking with them, they mention hope, love, understanding, and tolerance. Many know the AA prayer, "Let me accept the things I cannot change, give me courage to change the things I can change, and the wisdom to know the difference."

i) Expectations

Throughout history, unhappiness has been explained as a discrepancy between expectation and experience. If one expects more than one achieves, it is quite natural to feel badly.

Happiness is a state of harmony between you and the world around you. Every second is a small step of creation until the final fulfillment. This view will help set realistic expectations and avoid needless disappointment. Sometimes it is good to set relatively low goals and be happy with overachievement. After success and renewed confidence, one can set more ambitious goals.

One of the worst problems is lack of hope and confidence. Just say "I can do it," then try it and see how you do. You will likely get confidence that you can do more. If you are afraid of failure and don't even try, there is no chance for success. Visualize the positive, think positively, take a small step, then another small step, and surprise— you succeed.

Do you believe that over 80 you have fewer reasons to be happy and more reasons to be sad? What would be the result of such an attitude? Would it affect your health? Your self-confidence? Your activities? The amount of daily medications you take? Would it push you towards an alcoholic beverage to feel good? Would a negative outlook on life and a negative state of mind affect the mood of people close to you? Would that result in negative feedback? And what would be the consequence of all that?

If your expectations are negative, you could slip into a downward spiral, which many call aging. More likely, it is something else. You need to have realistic expectations. Winning the lottery is not realistic. Minor improvement in anything is realistic. Follow that up with another minor improvement, and another one, and another one.

Death is a realistic expectation. But does it have to be negative? You might just as well choose a positive attitude about the end of your life. Think of it as an accomplishment, as a fulfillment of your destiny.

Those who believe in a religion that promises Heaven after life will have a positive attitude. Those who see life as a biological, dynamic process involving thousands of generations in which you and every other link in the chain fulfills its role will also have a positive outlook on the last quintile of life.

Young people tend to worry about money, job, health, kids, education, and building a nest egg. "Keeping up with the Joneses" may be a concern. Despite these concerns and hard work and setbacks, there are many happy moments. They are usually busy, and one can easily see how they can feel happy about building their lives, their family, their company, and their nation.

Around age 50 to 55, the mortgage has been paid off, the kids are out of school, there may be a new house, and retirement is on the horizon. Then the older generation begins to pass away, and it becomes absolutely clear that life is not forever. Health problems multiply, and you begin to look at retirement not so much as a time to finally enjoy yourself, but as possibly signaling the end of life. Will the savings last?

The upward and downward trends in life are biologically and sociologically determined. How about your attitude, your mood, and your mental and physical health?

There is one simple way to make life's downhill slide the happiest time of your life: make it an uphill path. The magic word is better, better, and better! If you can, focus on the creation of life, the blossoming, the blooming, the bearing of fruit, and growth.

Be involved: work with children, help in social services, teach and share your wisdom and life experience. Make betterment a daily goal in anything you do. Work on your health, your lifestyle, sports, finance, and learning. Even keeping and caring for a pet is said to be therapeutic. Why? Because you are caring for a living being.

Even failures, mishaps, accidents, illnesses, and disasters have a positive side. It is a matter of how you look at it and what lessons are there for the future. Have you learned something? If a mistake is involved, will you try to not make that same mistake again? If it is just bad luck, that may be something you need to process as well. Not everything is under our control. How do we live knowing that so much is not under our control?

Betterment can be in the tiniest of steps. Walk for five minutes. After you accomplish that you may feel motivated to continue on. Often, motivation comes after one starts rather than before.

Step outside at night and look at the stars. Take a deep breath and think and feel grateful for just being alive. If you are so inclined say "Better, better, and better." Don't avoid the future but welcome it.

Have curiosity and wonder: How will it work out? Will my fears or my hopes be realized? What else will I experience and learn? If you acknowledge that you can't control much of what is coming, particularly since so much is unknowable, the task of the future is much more manageable

Particularly enjoy every sign of improvement, saying "Thank you."

j) Unhappiness and Depression

Everyone encounters problems that are commonly interpreted as reasons for unhappiness or depression. Financial problems, failure in job or career, family problems, health problems, loneliness, lack of respect, and much more. Surely, when you first encounter a problem, you don't feel happy about it. But working on a solution and finding one will make you feel good, successful, and even happy. Problems themselves are not unhappiness and are not only inevitable but the challenge of life.

Persistence of feeling bad may be an early reminder that you have veered away from the road of a safe and healthy life. It's a very useful gauge, like a low fuel gauge reading in your car. You need to refill your tank. Feeling bad should trigger an effort to feel better. The first step might be a conversation with yourself about the cause and timing of the episode of feeling bad.

Though it is completely normal to have an episode of feeling badly, if it persists for more than a couple of weeks and begins to affect everyday functioning, it may be something more severe. Particularly, if you start to feel "hopeless, helpless, and lost," it may be a clinical depression. Another warning sign is if you no longer get pleasure out of the things that usually do give you pleasure. Sleeping or eating too little or too much are also signs that things are amiss. If you also begin to question why you are alive or begin to think you would rather be dead, it is time to get help.

Help can be in various forms. If you are comfortable talking with your minister or primary care physician, that would be a good start. Otherwise, consult a mental health professional, a psychiatric social worker, clinical psychologist, or psychiatrist. Both psychotherapy and medication are often extremely helpful in providing relief. They are often used together.

Case example: During a recent vacation in Germany, I tried talking with a 95-year-old senior owner of a hotel, now managed by his son. He appeared to be quite healthy, fit, and friendly. I had seen him riding his bike and carrying a ladder to change a light bulb. He was also still driving a car, and I had seen him bumping into another car in his parking lot, without any damage. I knew his wife and sister had died six months ago, and I started to ask him about his health and if he was still in good shape and being happy. But whatever I asked, he answered by talking about his escape from the Luftwaffe after the German army collapsed. I asked about him hitting the other car, and he responded with the same story.

I then asked his son about his father's health. "Oh, he is in good health," he said, "but he ignores requests about taxes and legal inquiries. He locks everything up, we don't even get a key for his house. And we don't know what to do."

I asked how my co-author, Jay, would interpret this behavior, and he tells me this is likely a case of clinical depression with paranoid features. He could be helped by medication or electro convulsive therapy (ECT) even at his advanced age. The issue is his denial of there being a problem, refusal to go to a doctor or therapist, and the various laws that protect individuals from being coerced into treatment if they don't present an immediate threat to themselves or others.

The only conclusion I can think of, is that we should expect to be mentally incapacitated at some point and prepare for such a situation by keeping perfect order in our affairs, have a will, and put instructions and authorizations for our most trusted family members in writing while we are still healthy.

k) Tragedy and Other Problems

Finally, how can someone be happy if extreme tragedy strikes? About five percent of people in the USA are very poor, living on less than two dollars a day. How about being old, poor, and sick at the same time?

This book cannot cure financial or health problems per se. Instead, we hope to help you anticipate and avoid some serious problems and cope with them when they strike.

Two major reasons for extreme unhappiness are drug abuse and disrupted family relationships. These often appear together. Financial ruin often results. But even in the worst situations, there is a potential for going up or down. The basic steps to restoring health and happiness should be:

1. **Pray and meditate**. Take an honest and realistic inventory of your condition. Write it down. Tell yourself, it can get better. Imagine the light. Be assured, there is a way. Think positive. Rebuild your self-confidence. Package fear and bad habits in a box; throw the box into a river, and see it floating away.
2. **Get advice**. See a counselor. Talk to the pastor of your church and your doctor. If you can afford it, get personal counseling. If you know an attorney, any expert, your former boss, anybody with experience and wisdom, get advice.
3. **Clean up your finances.** Try to pay off your credit card balance if you can get a less expensive loan. Negotiate with your bank about a loan and payment terms. Rid yourself from useless commitments and responsibilities for others that are exacerbating the problems. Cleaning all your affairs, cleaning up your house, your desk, your car, your files, your relationships, and getting everything in picture-perfect order will have a very positive effect on your mental sanity.
4. **Live healthfully.** Breathe fresh air. Do whatever exercise you are able to do, even waving your arms, taking a few steps, and drink plenty of water. Eat light and healthy food. Wash up, clean the clutter, talk to yourself, smile, sing.

Here is an example of a real-world difficult scenario:

"I am 85 and my husband 87. I am diabetic, and 2 years ago I became 50 percent blind and lost my job as an accountant. I have severe back pain unless I take pain medication. My husband is relatively healthy, but alcohol-dependent and has been out of a job for the last 10 years. He is weak, had a car accident, lost his driver's license, and stays at home. My son is in prison; my daughter used to live with us until she got in a fight with my husband and he threw her out with her two kids, age 8 and 12. Her husband, whom she never married, disappeared years ago. She moved in with a friend, but they lost their apartment, and she is now homeless, living in a shelter, and I have taken the kids back. My husband is very aggressive and has threatened me with a knife on multiple occasions. He refuses to let our daughter live with us. I get social security of $1500 a month, my husband $2100, but he spends it all on alcohol. We took out a mortgage 8 years ago to pay for a treatment facility for my husband, but he quickly relapsed.

"Now we are behind on the mortgage. My car broke down; it is very old. I am very afraid of my husband. I have a sister in California, where I could live, but I feel responsible for the kids and my daughter. She just can't find any job, and I have supported her as much as I can, but now I am broke. I need a new car. I tried to get my husband into a retirement home, but he refuses. Our home is worth about $90,000 less the mortgage balance of $18,000.

"I went to get help at the township. A social worker tried to convince my husband to enter a treatment facility, but he later threatened me for arranging this. A friend urged me to divorce him and go live with my sister. But how about the kids? I am desperate, out of money, and afraid. I am trying to find a job, but I can hardly read."

The following is not meant to be a specific advice, but only an example how our general approach might be applied. It may be overly optimistic considering your health condition, and it requires work and research. Expect that only one out of five resources you explore will be acceptable. Don't be discouraged. You will definitely find the solutions and people that will help you.

1. Be confident that you will find a solution.

    a. Write down all pertinent facts about your finances.
        i. Cash
        ii. Mortgage
        iii. Income
        iv. Bills due now and future
        v. House value
        vi. Other assets
    b. Write down the list of problem areas to be attacked:
        i. Husband
        ii. Daughter
        iii. Bank
        iv. Kids
        v. Job
        vi. Health

    Close your eyes and pray or meditate and imagine a positive outcome.

2. Get advice

    See an attorney
    You must separate from your husband to prevent a terrible tragedy.
    Have divorce papers made and an action plan.
    Negotiate payment terms.

3. Attack the problem areas:

    a. Help your daughter to find a job, write a resume, dress up neatly, and go job hunting. Use computer help at the library.
    b. Find a job for yourself, even at minimum wage.
    c. Find a nursing home in your area for your husband. Keep all that secret. Fill out the application. He pays $30,000 down once the house is sold, plus sixty percent

of his SS check, and the rest is covered by Medicaid. Give the contract to your attorney.

d. Put your house on the market with the best real estate company.
e. Look for a car for about $8000, get rid of your old car. In the future, let your daughter do the driving.
f. Find an apartment for you, the kids, and your daughter. Set a rent budget of $1200 per month.
g. Your daughter may join if she contributes $800 for rent and half the household cost.
h. Show the bank your plans and negotiate a short-term loan of $5000. You may play hardball and threaten to default on the mortgage. But your plan must be sound, including your daughter's income, sale of your house, expenses, etc.
i. Once you have all forms and plans resolved, obtain an acceptable offer for your house, if that is possible without your husband's consent, let's say for $90,000, finalize all papers with your attorney and file for divorce. Move into your rented apartment without letting your husband know. The attorney will request a visit from your husband. The attorney will tell your husband that he will file criminal charges for aggravated assault with a deadly weapon if he threatens you again.
j. Your husband needs to agree to the divorce settlement and go to AA or other alcohol treatment facility.

All this needs to be done right now, as fast as possible. Find a friend that can help you, including driving you around.

4. Stay healthy:

   a. Visit your doctor and stay healthy yourself.
   b. Be extremely disciplined on nutrition and a healthy lifestyle with your new family.
   c. Use all available resources and services from Medicaid, food stamps, housing support, childcare support, and township. Your doctor, township, and library will help with advice.

d. Pay back your mortgage, credit card balance, attorney bill and bank loan. Put the surplus into an investment account.

Will it work? I don't know. But it's a plan worth fighting for.

11. Religion

Can religion help us live a happy and healthy life? When our survival depended on the kindness of gods who ruled over storms, floods, sun, diseases, birth and death, it was vital to keep the gods friendly. Worshippers paid tribute and respect in the form of sacrifices and worship. Still today, farmhouses in Saxon regions have wooden heads of horses mounted on the roof as a sign of respect to the god Thor (Thursday) or Donar (Donnerstag in German) who would ride his horse through the air throwing thunder (Donner in German) and lightning bolts.

It was not lack of science or understanding of natural forces that made people believe in gods. It was the uncertainty about life-threatening events.

What caused the demise of the gods? Their sheer multiplicity was their undoing. The in-fighting and power plays among the gods created the potential for a more powerful godly dictator that could rule over all nature. A single god that was more powerful than Wotan, Thor, or Donar. The new, all powerful, one-god religions offered better insurance against the uncertainties of life.

When astronomers like Galileo and Copernicus explained the heavenly bodies, and when Darwin contradicted creationism, philosophers trashed religions as myths and, not surprisingly, atheists have grown in numbers ever since.

However, it is also true that today, when natural phenomenon are easily explained by chemistry, mathematics, physics, and biology, there are still many believers in religion. Even the very origin of life seems understandable. Evolution explains much as well. Nonetheless, uncertainty in every day persists, and God seems necessary to many.

But what is the benefit? When Real Madrid plays Juventus Torino, they pray to win and so does Juventus. But one team loses. We may pray that the stock market rises, but God just won't listen. We all know that there is no guarantee. Not in soccer, cancer, love, or business. Or is there? Praying is cheap, and why not bet on all the horses in the race?

The clerics do their best to keep believers loyal with stories of miracles, promises of an afterlife, and punishment for sinners.

Churches are convenient assembly places of the community. Like the Ting, the meeting place every Tuesday (=Tingsday) under a big oak tree thousands of years ago, people find advice, help, consolation, encouragement, and hope. And if hope heals hopelessness and gives peace and even happiness, even a devoted atheist might admit that religion has some value for those that practice it.

Still, that does not explain why millions of people in all countries believe in God and pray. People should have long noticed that when you pray for rain, it is a hit-and-miss proposition. If religions have existed as long as humans, religion must offer more than a myth explaining natural phenomena.

My physics teacher in high school predicted that one day people would explore space and step on the moon. We discussed the physics of the universe, and the great teacher said with a somber voice, "Where science ends, God begins."

I raised the question: Does that mean, when science advances, God retreats?

He was a bit confused and stated, "That is up to each believer."

I dared to oppose: If there is a God, he (or she) cannot be a mythical figure in heaven but can only be a force among us and within us and thus become greater with each discovery.

Ironically, atheists, wellness fans, and psychologists have expanded on this: meditation and prayer are one way of programming our subconscious. And our subconscious usually overrides rational thinking and planning. It is not science killing religion, but science revealing the core secret of religion.

The problem with religion may not be the apocalypse of the gods, but the poor presentation by the churches. It was not Darwin against God, but Darwin against clerics that were afraid of losing in the needless contest of science versus God.

Already, we have discovered the creation process within living cells. The probability of no other life on distant planets is next to zero. We have a problem imagining certain things that overwhelm our tiny and short human view. We cannot imagine Nothing or Eternity. We have discovered the Big Bang, but what was there before the Big Bang? What caused it? An accident, when the eternal sea of Nothing collapsed. Was that God?

It may be considered blasphemy, but it is irrelevant to know for sure if there is a God who created life and the universe. It only matters if there is belief— and that belief helps us deal with life and its uncertainty. In that way, prayer may help in a soccer match. Or help us to live longer? Or die in peace?

12. Facing the End

So far, this book has prepared us for a pleasant last quintile of our life. Now let's go a step beyond. No matter how lucky or successful we are in building and living the last twenty years, there will be a point when we realize that the end is near. Let's assume we live happily to age 100, and after a great birthday party, we have trouble getting up from our chair. We could not recognize several old friends, we have balance problems and need a cane or walker, and we have vision problems and are not allowed to drive a car. After 100 yards of walking around the block, we give up. No chance to join a tennis game or swim laps.

This is the endgame. Is it possible to make these months or years enjoyable and even productive?

Productive? Yes, we can be a model or ideal for younger generations, providing an example of successful aging. We can pass along what we learned over our long lives.

Enjoy? Yes, although now our life will be quite different. There are various ways to happiness in the endgame. The key is envisioning it clearly and making plans while our brain still works well. Happiness starts with realistic expectations.

We need to find help, starting with daily assistance at home or in a facility. This help includes personal care involving all bodily functions like toileting, bathing, eating, walking, getting in and out of bed, or even turning on the television.

Another helper should be available to assist with financial affairs, organizing transportation, medical services, and legal projects.

Another very helpful service is mental training. Most facilities for the elderly will offer group mental stimulation. Games or activities like reading aloud, watching movies, and group discussions are an enjoyable way to keep minds alive and awake. Browsing through memories, writings, letters, and albums are stimulating and enjoyable activities. Writing articles, books, your biography, letters, or notes in a diary is a wonderful and productive activity.

More practical things like updating hearing aids, eyeglasses, walker, wheelchair, laptop or tablet, or even shoes and clothing are important. Basically, make sure everything offers maximum comfort and functionality.

Traveling with friends or paid companion to parks, exhibitions, theater, or just to watching the sunset on a beach can make your life worthwhile.

Avoiding scam artists is another challenge. Your trusted friends, relatives, attorney, and helpers need to protect you. It would be wonderful if your son, daughter, your spouse, or your best friend could be your most trusted helper and coordinator for all services. Even if part of their motivation is inheriting your wealth, that is okay. Your personal attorney or legal and financial advisor should keep an eye on inheritance hunters and structure your will in such a way that it protects you and your loved ones.

But now the end is near. Will we panic? Will we live in fear? Will we make irrational decisions?

Rule number one, like in all catastrophes, is not to make things worse. It can always get worse, even when one is close to death; or it can get better. The difference is small. Panicking or living in fear will increase stress and not only shorten life but also promote sickness and suffering.

How can we make things better? How can we convert the fear of death into a positive attitude? It is certainly a new challenge, one that we have never faced before. Think about how we dealt with new challenges in the past?

Throughout our lives, from learning to walk, going to pre-school, reading, making friends, playing games or sports, graduating from every level of school, obtaining a job, moving and finding new friends, marrying, having children, buying a house, and surviving illnesses, it was always a new challenge.

So how will we fare? Are we going to successfully cope or fail miserably? No one knows for sure, but there is something increasingly true as we age: we have a track record.

One way to face uncertainties is to look back. Play back your memory of how you faced and overcame previous crises and challenges.

You might say "But I never faced a challenge with a certain negative outcome. I never died before."

Partly true, but many things that turned out well were also new challenges. Again, the purpose of this book is not to allow you live 200 years, but to make the last phase of your life pleasant as opposed to miserable. So, the memory of successfully managing past challenges will be very comforting in facing the next one.

Another way of accepting an unavoidable disaster is to practice the AA prayer:

God, grant me the serenity to accept the things I cannot change, Courage to change the things I can, and wisdom to know the difference.

Then you may ask: "But I don't have a choice? I can't change destiny. What can I do?"

Yes, you do have a choice; you can make things a whole lot worse. Here is how:

Stop caring. "Who cares? What's the point? Life will be over soon." House, health, finances, let everything go to hell! Get drunk. You will surely experience misery.

On the other hand, if you have to die tomorrow, have the gutters fixed today, get a landscaper, check your finances, your will, and get things in order. Get a haircut. Get a helper to clean the attic and the garage. Then lay down, fold your hands, and smile.

A very intelligent retired scientist did all that for his terminally ill wife. He had always taken care of her, and he continued to do so as they both aged. Then the surprise. He got a stroke and passed away before she did. Now she was totally helpless, did not know their finances, their medical information, how to start the computer, or any passwords. She didn't know about the will, cemetery, and funeral arrangements. Neither she nor he had prepared rationally for the end.

It might be a good idea for all of us to write down the information our heirs and loved ones might need in the days and months after our death. Whether that be a listing of computer and online passwords or a description of assets and obligations or even just a favorite recipe, please write it down for those who have come to count on you for that information. You will not be around forever, and the end might be like much of life: unanticipated.

When we see people die, we cry, we miss a life-long companion, we feel sympathy, sorrow, and we know that this ultimate disaster will happen to us. Funerals help us say goodbye to loved ones but remind us of what is coming. We must make a conscious effort to change our attitude from terror to a realistic understanding about death in order to live in harmony with life from beginning to end. The "end of life" is actually not the end, but birth and death are both parts of life. Life is both "hello" and "goodbye."

We have learned that death is a natural process and integral to life itself. We understand that it is fulfilment. Those who believe in Heaven or an afterlife will consider the exit as an entrance to eternal life. We can also be sure that we live on spiritually in the minds of those who know and love us. And we can set an example for our spouse and offspring in the way we cross the river Hades.

13. The End

All the while, things will progress more or less rapidly. Suddenly or slowly, certain organs and physical parts of the body will begin to fail. Arthritis causes pain with every move. The digestive system malfunctions. Your memory deteriorates, and you sometimes don't recognize your closest relatives. You can't read. There can be all kinds of scenarios.

Doctors and your family expect that the end is near. You rest. You have made provisions for your passing away, possibly donated your body to science and have signed papers to disconnect life support if family and doctor agree. You may get hospice care. If in pain, you get pain medicine to make you feel better. You get visits from friends and family. You may stop eating. You feel and enjoy the last handshake. And one day or night, your heart simply stops.

There are scenarios where you are suffering badly and are quite aware that there is no cure, and you are a burden for your family. You want to end your life. Unfortunately, our law and culture puts limits on that, but you can ask for medications that will reduce your suffering, letting you rest peacefully without pain, allowing nature to do the rest.

At least nine states have de-criminalized doctor-assisted ending of life for terminally ill patients. The rules are quite detailed and specific. Under these laws, the patient would self-administer a prescribed drug.

If you have learned throughout this book and throughout life to understand and have a realistic relationship with life, biologically and philosophically, the process of envisioning and planning this last chapter of your life should be a normal and pleasant exercise.

However well prepared for, the end stage of life nonetheless may be difficult. "In what way exactly is life great," you would ask, "when your body falls apart piece-by-piece, and one by one, all your friends die?"[16]

Back to nature. You have been a productive element of the human species. Elephants know it, cats know it, your doctor knows it, and you know it. Peace is near. The end is here.

You have decided upon the extent of life support.

You have no fear. You feel no more pain. Someone is holding your hand. Are your loved ones there? The hand feels good. You are not alone.

Your memory plays back images of your life. Do you smile?

You are handed family pictures. Someone had the foresight of printing a photobook. Was it you? The pictures are fuzzy. But the images become brighter.

You remember one close friend, the one, to whom you could always talk, and who always gave you advice. Perhaps you had lost contact, but now, you see, you feel, you hear the voice, "I love you, come, let's go, I am here with you." You have arrived.

Further Reading

https://www.deathwithdignity.org/learn/end-of-life-resources/

https://www.compassionandchoices.org/

Part II: the Aging Brain

Not only our body, but our brain is aging. Is aging preventable? What causes aging? Can aging be slowed? Part II of this book explains how cells reproduce, age, and eventually die. It also explains how DNA, the reproductive program stored in each cell, works to maximize longevity and health. However, DNA changes by accidental mutation, with exposure to cancerous chemicals, by radiation, and as a result of old age. More recently, we have learned that many more factors influence DNA. Things like physical and mental exercises may preserve cellular DNA better than any medicine. There are other surprises. For example, sleep provides a nightly cleaning service for the brain. Who would have thought that we have some control about how our brain ages? Let's get into the details.

In part II of this book, Jay M Pomerantz, MD, provides an overview of the latest research about the link between the mind to the brain and both to the body, particularly as it relates to old age. Dr. Pomerantz practiced clinical psychiatry for almost 50 years and treated a variety of patients including the old and very old, from which he learned much about the underlying brain mechanisms that so adversely affected many of his patients.

Now over age 80, he teaches neuroscience at Temple University's Osher Lifelong Learning Institute (OLLI). He is particularly interested in what neuroscience tells us about the aging brain and the possibilities for keeping it functioning optimally.

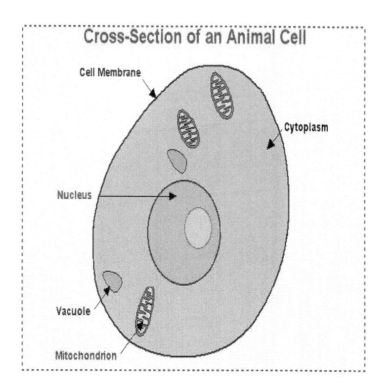

The cell is the basic functional unit of the human body. It is the building block, a self-contained and fully operational living entity. There are about 200 different kinds of specialized cells in the human body.

One type of specialized cell is the neuron, and it is the key to brain function. It both sends and receives signals from other neurons in the nervous system, thereby providing a two-way connection between the brain and the rest of the body. Neurons and their connections, called synapses, are the building blocks of the brain.

1. The Brain of a Sea Slug

Neuroscientist Eric R. Kandel[17] looked at the sea slug (aphysia) 50 years ago and saw a 3-pound animal whose simple nervous system, with 30 thousand neurons as compared to the human brain's 100 billion neurons, might be a great tool to begin understanding brain mechanisms, especially memory. Kandel's studies revealed that all animals, including humans, learn by strengthening synapses, the connections between neurons. Long-term memory involves not only strengthening synapses but building new ones. Repeated use of a particular synapse sends a message to the nuclei of the involved neurons to physically grow new connections (synapses) between the communicating neurons.

That means that brains are "plastic," constantly changing, adding, and strengthening synapses with use and weakening or even losing them with disuse. The neuroscientist's credo is "Neurons that fire together, wire together." Like the rest of the body, the brain strengthens with active use and atrophies with disuse. More particularly, brain circuits responsible for specific activities and specific memories get more robust with use and dwindle away with inactivity.

Each human neuron supports approximately 10,000 synaptic connections, resulting in approximately 100 trillion synapses. That's where our memory and ability to work with words, facts, thoughts, feelings, motor activities, and plans reside. Also, synapses and their affiliated brain circuits manage our subconscious maintenance of vital functions such as controlling blood pressure, breathing, and heart rate.

These discoveries, for which Kandel shared the 2000 Nobel Prize in Physiology or Medicine with Arvid Carlsson of Goeteborg University in Sweden and Paul Greengard of the Rockefeller University, provide evidence for the "connectionist" view of the brain as a highly plastic organ defined by interlaced connections among neurons and brain regions. Each brain is unique and defines the person. Even identical twins are quite different, particularly as their brains re-model in different ways over time. It would not be incorrect to state: "you are your synapses."

Schematic of Nerve Cells and Synapses

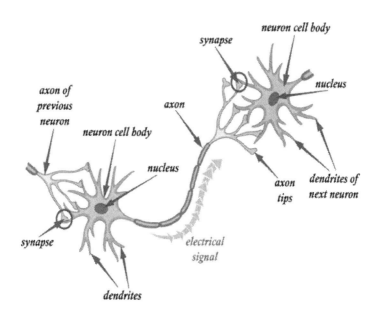

2. The Memory of a Taxi Driver

London cab drivers in training spend three to four years driving around the city on mopeds, memorizing a labyrinth of 25,000 streets within a 10-kilometer radius of Charing Cross train station, as well as thousands of tourist attractions and hot spots. "The "knowledge," as it is called, is unique to London taxi licensing and involves a series of grueling exams that only about 50 percent of hopefuls pass. Postulating that such training might show up in structural MRI's (a brain scan), licensed London taxi drivers, were analyzed and compared with control subjects who did not drive taxis. The hippocampus is the area of the brain that is associated with memory and spatial navigation. The posterior hippocampi of taxi drivers were significantly larger relative to those of non-taxi driver subjects. In addition, a more anterior hippocampal region was larger in non-taxi driver subjects than in taxi drivers. Hippocampal volume correlated with the amount of time spent as a taxi driver (positively in the posterior and negatively in the anterior hippocampus).

These data fit what is known from other studies: the posterior hippocampus stores spatial representations of the environment and can expand to accommodate new knowledge. It is clear that there is a capacity for specific plastic changes in the structure of the healthy adult human brain in response to environmental demands.[18]

Although it might be argued that people with initial big posterior hippocampi choose to become taxi drivers because they are good at geography, a follow up study of trainees before, during and after licensing showed that it was the training process that caused the growth in the brain. One can produce profound changes in the brain with training.

3.   Muscle Memory

Muscle memory (athletes talk about this all the time) exists, although the name is a misnomer. A better name might be "subconscious memory." It is the information stored in the brain, most readily accessible—or only accessible—by non-conscious means. These partially or fully automatic functions are handled through the brain's connections to the rest of the nervous system and through spinal cord and peripheral nerve relays to our muscles and the other organs, glands, and tissues. Blood pressure, heart rate, and release of stress and other hormones are all monitored and controlled by the brain, usually without our being consciously aware of what's going on.

4. Teaching an Old Dog New Tricks

Brain Plasticity in Older Individuals

For a long time, it had been assumed that brain plasticity peaks at young age and then gradually decreases as one gets older. Thus, the expression that "one cannot teach an old dog new tricks," implying that older people who have become used to doing things in a particular way cannot easily abandon their habits or change their behavior. Now, thanks to advances in medical imaging techniques for the assessment of brain structure and function, there is mounting evidence for lifelong brain plasticity.

New motor and other skills can be acquired at any age even though progress may be somewhat slower in older as compared to younger populations. The importance of these results should not be underestimated. We live in a highly dynamic society in which change proceeds at a rapid pace. These phenomena require successful individuals to abandon their pre-existing old habits and replace them with new ones, continuously challenging the adaptability and flexibility of their brains.

Given the steadily increasing proportion of older adults, evidence for lifelong brain plasticity is hopeful for society in general. However, older adults need to accept the challenge and adapt to new contexts. This will help counter the negative consequences of another process, age-related brain degeneration, such as loss of neurons, synapses, and brain circuits, as individuals age. [19]

5. Old Mice Getting Younger

A recent mouse study suggests that the increasing difficulty in learning new information and skills that most of us experience as we age is not necessarily due to difficulty in acquiring new information. Instead, much of the problem may be too much information of a similar kind accumulated over the years. Weakening the unwanted or out-of-date connections is as important as making new connections.

To the researchers' surprise, old mice were found to be good at making new strong connections but showed an impaired ability to weaken existing connections. The resulting overload of similar information produces internal conflict. Bear in mind that each mouse neuron, like a human neuron, has thousands of potential points of contact (i.e., synapses), and you will see the importance of turning down the noise. [20]

In the extreme, how can you reliably remember where you last parked your car if you equally remember all the places where you parked it previously?

6. Dementia

Losses and Defects of Brain Cells

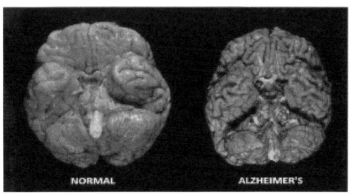

Pictures of Two Human Brains

Even as we age, the normal aging brain continues to look much as throughout adult life. That is certainly not true if the individual suffers from a dementing disease like Alzheimer's. Dementia is a broad term that refers to deficits in thinking or memory that impair a person's ability to perform everyday functions. To receive a diagnosis of dementia, a person must experience deficits beyond what is expected from a normal course of aging. The most common form of dementia is Alzheimer's Disease. Other brain diseases, such as Vascular Dementia, Lewy Body Dementia, Parkinson's, Frontotemporal Dementia, and others can also result in dementia. In persons with dementia, the brain changes relatively quickly, over a few years, into a shrunken, scarred, dysfunctional shell of itself. In fact, the Alzheimer's brain shrinks down to as little as one-third its normal size as the disease progresses.

If the Alzheimer brain looks grossly bad, its function is even worse. Memory, especially short-term memory, is quickly compromised with the rest of the brain's function soon following suit.

Microscopically, one can see that the neurons are surrounded and killed by an accumulation of toxic protein plaques known as amyloid beta, and the neurons themselves are destroyed from within by another toxic protein conjugate, tau tangles.

These toxic proteins seem to figure prominently in the disease, but there is no consensus about why and how they appear. Are they of infectious origin, predetermined by genes, the product of inefficient removal of cellular waste products, or related to immune hyperactivity? Is it a combination of several of these factors or something else entirely?

In the early years of the 21st century, the pharmaceutical industry bet billions on experimental drugs that cleared the amyloid plaques, but the resultant gains in brain function were minimal, and the effort is now mostly abandoned. Other researchers are busy chasing the tau tangles and other leads. However, at this point, Alzheimer's and most other dementias remain resistant to treatment. That being said, there are some interesting possibilities for delaying or possibly preventing Alzheimer's and other dementing illnesses that we will explore shortly.

Whereas all of us, as we get older, may become a bit forgetful, perhaps occasionally losing our car keys, the Alzheimer sufferer, even when finding the keys no longer remembers what they are for— or even how the key is useful in starting the car! Eventually, the spouse and other close family members are forgotten. The course is variable, but eventually leads to greater and greater brain dysfunction, ending in an inability to feed oneself or even swallow. Death comes too slowly for all concerned as personhood is lost with progressive brain dysfunction.

The statistics are grim when we consider the increasing steep rise in the likelihood of Alzheimer's and other dementing neurological diseases over time, especially in the last quintile of possible life.

7. Dementia Prevalence by Age Groups

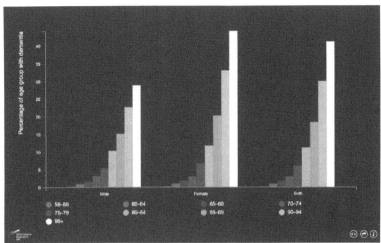

Prevalence of Dementia by Age in Males, Females, and Overall

As one can see in the above chart, dementia, including Alzheimer's, Fronto-Temporal Disease, Lewy Body Disease, Vascular Dementia, Parkinson's, etc., rises precipitously with age. At 90-94 years, it has a prevalence of over 30 percent in females and over 20 percent in males. At 95+, the prevalence rises to 45 percent in females and to almost 30 percent in males.

Females are more likely to get dementia than males in every age cohort. That goes against the usual health trends in which females are usually advantaged, resulting in their living longer on average than males.

8. Preventing Dementia?

Enhancing Cognitive Reserve

There are some intriguing studies that suggest that although medical scientists do not have a cure or even agreement on what causes age-related brain diseases, certain prevention strategies may be helpful. We will discuss each of these possible preventives in some detail, presenting some of the underlying scientific evidence.

A number of studies have examined how participation in mentally stimulating activities throughout life can protect cognitive function (ability to think, remember, and plan) in older age through impacting cognitive reserve. Verghese and colleagues[21] studied whether participation in leisure activities reduced the risk of dementia in community-residing older adults. The authors found that leisure activities such as reading, playing board games, playing musical instruments, and dancing were all associated with a reduced risk of developing dementia.

In a long-term study involving the same individuals over a period of years, researchers documented an association between engagement in mentally-stimulating activities and the degree of cognitive decline experienced over time. Wilson and colleagues[22] reported on a cohort of 4,000 community-residing older adults. More frequent cognitive activity was associated with reduced cognitive decline during follow-up. Specifically, a one-point increase in the cognitive activity score was associated with an approximate 19 percent decrease in the annual rate of cognitive decline. The authors concluded that frequent participation in cognitively stimulating activities is associated with reduced cognitive decline in older persons.

Fritsch and colleagues[23] examined the relationship between participation in novelty-seeking leisure activities and the risk for developing Alzheimer's Disease (AD). By using a study method where each study participant was matched with someone otherwise similar in age, gender, and medical history, they compared AD patients with a control group of neighbors and friends of the cases plus a randomly selected group of community members. The odds of developing AD were lower among those who participated in activities involving an exchange of ideas. In addition, the odds of developing AD were even lower for those who frequently participated in novelty-seeking activities. They concluded that participation in a variety of mental activities across the life span may lower one's chances of developing AD.

Collectively, there is evidence that higher cognitive functioning in late adulthood is associated with a lifelong pursuit of complex cognitive activities. However, the studies reviewed above only show that the phenomena appear together in nature. That by itself, suggests but does not prove the causal role of cognitive activity.[24]

9. The Nun Study

It was 1991, and David Snowden sat across from a 100-year-old nun named Sister Mary, administering a psychological test. He asked her to remember a list of words, to draw geometric shapes, and she passed each exam while she talked and laughed, constantly aware.

After Sister Mary's death at 102, a lab examined her brain. She had been alert and without memory loss, but instead of looking at a healthy brain, scientists saw one riddled with visible knots of protein— an indication of full-blown Alzheimer's disease. Sister Mary was part of a very large research project on Alzheimer's called the Nun Study.[25]

It is a decades-long investigation of aging and brain health that followed 678 Catholic nuns living in School Sisters of Notre Dame convents across the United States. The sisters all agreed to open medical and personal records, undergo annual testing, and donate their brains after death. Because they had such similar routines, they presented a rare controlled opportunity to study aging without many of the complicating effects of environment — a "natural experiment."

One sample observation: Sister Bernadette never showed any signs of mental decay. She once guessed the time within four minutes without looking at a clock, while other sisters her age couldn't tell morning from night. But after she died of a heart attack at 85, an autopsy showed that her brain was riddled with the plaques and tangles of Alzheimer's.

"It was as if her neocortex (the part of the human brain involved in sensory perception, generation of motor commands, spatial reasoning, conscious thought, and language) was resistant to destruction for some reason," writes David Snowden, the epidemiologist who started the Nun Study and wrote "Aging with Grace," a book about the research. "Sister Bernadette appears to have been what we, and others, have come to call an 'escapee.' Death had intervened before her symptoms had time to surface."

In movies, media, and real life, dementia can seem inevitable, even demonic: it latches onto sufferers randomly and never relents until the mind is destroyed. The biological reality is much more complicated. Some people with mild cognitive impairment progress rapidly to full-blown Alzheimer's, while others trundle on indefinitely with only minor difficulties. A few even get better.

Autopsies of elderly people confirm that variability. In most Alzheimer's victims, cognitive problems are determined by the severity of the plaques and tangles in their brains. But some, like another nun, named Sister Maria, suffer profound declines yet are later found to have only early-stage Alzheimer's changes.

Others are Sister Bernadettes. Research suggests that perhaps a quarter of elderly adults who appear cognitively intact are harboring the pathological criteria for Alzheimer's. A third of Snowden's nuns were such "escapees," and recent analysis has found that 12 percent of Nun Study participants with the severest level of brain damage were not classified as "demented," though they might have been sliding into memory loss before death.

The participating nuns shared written accounts of their lives and personal essays from when they first took their vows with researchers, and these turned out to provide possible clues to the disease. Snowden found that sisters who wrote more complex personal essays in their youth tended not to develop the disease.

What accounts for this variability between brain pathology and symptoms? One possibility is what is termed "cognitive reserve." Those who use their brain more intensely over a lifetime may have many alternate neuronal circuits. When one pathway fails, there are others that are still available to retrieve the specific memory or do the specific task.

10. Physical Exercise

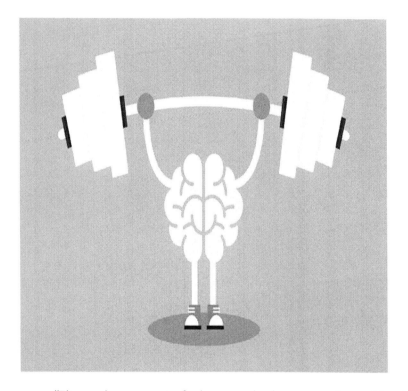

"The real reason we feel so good when we get our blood pumping is that it makes the brain function at its best," says John J. Ratey, author of *Spark: The Revolutionary New Science of Exercise and the Brain*. "The point of exercise is to build and condition the brain."

The reverse is also true: "What virtually no one recognizes," he warns, "is that inactivity is killing our brains."

"We now know that the brain is flexible, or *plastic*, in the parlance of neuroscientists— more Play-Doh than porcelain," Ratey explains. Our brains are constantly growing, and they can even be rewired. And exercise is the key.

Scientists understand that physical activity stresses our brains just as it stresses our muscles to force each system to rebuild more robustly. Neurons break down, then recover and become stronger and more resilient. "Aerobic exercise can change the brain's anatomy, physiology — and function," says New York University neural science professor Wendy Suzuki, PhD, author of *Healthy Brain, Happy Life*.

11. The Spark Plugs in our Brain

"Exercise is potent," Ratey goes on. "More nerve cells fire when we're exercising than when we're doing anything else. This activates the brain as a whole. It especially turns on arousal, attention, and executive functioning areas of the brain. That includes paying attention, organizing, planning, staying on task, understanding different points of view, regulating emotions, and keeping track of what you are doing.

The mechanism whereby exercise accomplishes this phenomenon involves neurotransmitters, chemicals that control synaptic communication. One such neurotransmitter is norepinephrine, which sparks attention, perception, motivation, and arousal; another is serotonin, which influences mood, impulsivity, anger, and aggression; and still another neurotransmitter is dopamine, which governs attention and learning, plus the sense of contentment and reward.

As our body moves, the brain learns how to move better the next time. Exercise also stimulates the cerebellum, which coordinates all the body's motor movements, like standing upright, hitting a tennis ball, or even walking a forest trail.

The prefrontal cortex is the brain's CEO; it's in charge of executive functions, controlling physical actions, receiving input, and issuing instructions to the body. Managing short-term working memory, judging, and planning are also its responsibility.

"When we exercise, particularly if the exercise requires complex motor movement, we're also exercising the area of the brain involved in the full suite of cognitive functions," Ratey explains. "We're causing the brain to repetitively fire signals along the same network of cells, which solidifies their connections."

The functions of learning and memory are concentrated in the hippocampus, a small region tucked in the brain's center. But we wouldn't be able to learn without input from the prefrontal cortex.

Exercise also stimulates neurotrophins, which build and maintain the brain's basic cell circuitry. Key among these neurotrophins is the recently discovered brain-derived neurotrophic factor (BDNF), a protein that incites neuron growth, particularly in important memory centers like the hippocampus.

"BDNF works in many ways," Ratey explains. "It makes brain cells work better; it grows them; it prevents them from eroding; it helps deal with stress; it provides the right environment for brain cells to prosper." BDNF is released when neurons fire, causing the brain to produce more BDNF. When we exercise, those neurons fire like crazy, elevating BDNF levels.

Physical activity also prompts other hormone factors into action: Insulin-like growth factor (IGF-1), vascular endothelial growth factor, and fibroblast growth factor all work with BDNF to enhance the molecular machinery of learning. In addition, the hormone IGF-1 delivers the brain's primary fuel — glucose — to neurons to spur learning.

Using magnetic resonance imaging (MRI), researchers discovered that BDNF helps the brain create new neurons from brain stem cells, a process called neurogenesis, in two crucial regions: the hippocampus, which is essential for long-term memory, and the olfactory bulb, the area responsible for smell and taste.

In tests on rodents, exercise *doubled* the rate of neurogenesis in the hippocampus, researcher Wendy Suzuki[26] reports. Plus, exercise increased the number of dendritic spines on the neurons as well as their length — all of which improve neuronal communication.

These physiological changes are called long-term potentiation (LTP), and in further rodent studies, researchers found that exercise-induced LTP improved hippocampal function as measured by a broad range of memory tests.

Other studies have shown similar memory gains for people. In a 2016 report published in *Frontiers in Human Neuroscience*, researchers conducted MRI scans on cross-country runners and identified "significantly greater connectivity" between parts of their brains associated with attention, decision-making, multitasking, processing sensory input, and memory, compared with a control group of nonrunners.[27]

To put it simply, exercise stimulates the brain in multiple ways, and produces significant advantages over a sedentary lifestyle, even beyond the obvious physical benefits.

12. Keeping the Brain Young

All the processes that physical activity induces in the brain add up to one conclusion: exercise helps keep our brains young and helps prevent cognitive decline as we age. It is the most important lifestyle change for anyone seeking to prevent the brain from deteriorating over time.

"Exercise not only makes our brains stronger, it also protects them. Physical activity induces the brain to create enzymes that chew up the amyloid beta-protein plaque that triggers Alzheimer's by strangling neurons," explains Harvard neurology professor Rudolph Tanzi, PhD, coauthor of *Super Brain*, a *New York Times* bestseller.

Another study by Tanzi's research team suggests that exercise also battles inflammation in the brain. A basic immune-system response to injury, inflammation can become chronic as we age, and studies have identified it as a primary agent in Alzheimer's. Exercise, along with lifestyle changes such as solid nutrition and good sleep, may actually help reverse Alzheimer's and cognitive decline.

The bottom line is the following: you have the power to change your brain. Start by lacing up your sneakers![28]

Another mechanism whereby exercise affects the brain has just been discovered. Exercise triggers the release of osteocalcin, a hormone manufactured by bone cells, and osteocalcin has a positive effect on memory. Studies[29] done in the Columbia University laboratory of Gerard Karsenty examined a role for osteocalcin in age-related memory loss and revealed that memory loss in aged mice could be improved by infusions of osteocalcin. The same improvements (i.e. improved performance in memory tests) were seen when blood plasma from young mice, which is rich in osteocalcin, was injected into aged mice. Conversely, depletion of osteocalcin in plasma from young mice (using specific anti-osteocalcin antibodies) eliminated the memory-improving effects.

Do these findings suggest that exercise, both mental and physical, can prevent or even reverse the benign memory loss associated with normal aging? That answer is a resounding yes, especially when combined with some other preventatives that we will discuss shortly.

Can exercise prevent or reverse Alzheimer's? Probably not, but it's good to know that even moderate exercise, such as walking, might delay things a bit. The Nun Study also suggests that cognitive reserve developed over a lifetime of learning and intensely using one's brain might mitigate and delay some of the symptoms even as the disease destroys neurons and synapses.

Mental and physical exercise are not the only tools available to protect our brains from getting "functionally old" even as we age chronologically. Let's now consider some exciting new research about the purpose of sleep.

13. The Importance of Sleep

Neuroscientist Jeff Iliff,[30] now working at Oregon Health & Science University, was a part of a University of Rochester Medical Center team that discovered a remarkable brain-cleansing system.

Sleep, particularly deep sleep, allows our brains to flush out toxic waste. The waste products are byproducts of metabolism and cell death. This waste, including the Alzheimer's-linked protein, amyloid beta, builds up in our brains during the day. If not cleared during sleep, some researchers go as far as to say that the Alzheimer's, Parkinson's, and other chronic brain diseases result.

Illif postulates that sleep has evolved to maximize maintenance-type functions in our brain, and this cleaning process is just one of them. It's arguably not even the most important one. In any event, our brain function is optimized when housekeeping functions happen during sleep. Sufficient sleep allows us to maximize our performance while we're awake.

It turns out that cerebrospinal fluid (CSF), the fluid that surrounds the brain, has another major function besides cushioning the brain. Illif concludes: "We were able to show that a substantial portion of CSF is actually recirculating back into and through the brain. It does this by essentially using the blood vessels as a scaffold to provide access to the entire brain tissue. The movement of this fluid along vessels and through the spaces between the brain's cells appears to be involved in the clearance of amyloid beta and other toxic waste products out of the brain's interstitial fluid."

Furthermore, Illif's group showed that this cleaning process is primarily a feature of the sleeping brain. Both the movement of cerebrospinal fluid along the outside of blood vessels and back through the brain, and the clearance of amyloid beta, occur much more rapidly in a naturally sleeping and anesthetized brain, compared to the waking brain.

They also went on to study both aging and injured mouse brains and learned that the cleaning process during sleep slows down.

The Paul G. Allen Family Foundation is funding Illif's group to extend the work on sleep and the aging brain from mouse models into humans. The first step in that process is to develop clinical imaging approaches to measure the system's activity in the sleeping and waking human brain. The study will then move on to analyze that process in the aged human brain and in the brains of people who appear to have the beginnings of Alzheimer's disease.

That's really exciting and promising for the future. This sleep-cleaning system may be a new therapeutic target, and imaging it may allow diagnosis at an earlier stage in the disease process.[31]

14. Telomeres

Those of us lucky enough to arrive at age 80 and beyond understand that the aim is not just living longer but living well during that time. Quality of life is paramount. Delaying the development of disease and disability, mental or physical, is crucial. Or, if diseases do appear, minimizing their effect is important. If one can stay disease-free or well treated until relatively old age, there is another important benefit. The end stage is likely short, and there is usually a relatively good death.

These issues and others are discussed at length in a 2017 book, "The Telomere Effect" by Dr. Elizabeth Blackburn, a molecular biologist, who won the Nobel Prize in Medicine (2009). Her co-author is Dr. Elissa Epel, a psychologist whose research focuses on chronic stress and aging.

They talk about "healthspan" versus "diseasespan" and define those as extending the duration of the time feeling well and healthy (healthspan) versus the time spent feeling ill and compromised (diseasespan).

Blackburn and Epel approach the issue of having more health and less disease by emphasizing the capacity for cellular renewal. Most of our cells, not only in the body but in parts of the brain, can regenerate and curtail premature aging. However, aging or stressed cells leak— they release what are called "pro-inflammatory" substances, such as cytokines, that results in chronic inflammation throughout the body.

Chronic inflammation builds plaques in our cardiac and cerebral arteries, eats away at pancreas cells, which renders us diabetic, and halt the regulation of immune functions. A dysfunctional immune system may not react to early cancers until it is too late. A dysfunctional overactive immune system characterized by chronic inflammation is also associated with and, possibly the cause of, a variety of mental conditions, especially major depression.

Blackburn and Epel suggest that the end caps on our cellular chromosomal DNA, the telomeres, are similar to the plastic tips of shoelaces. When the caps are intact, cellular division is freer of unwanted events like slowing cell division or stimulating the creation of cancer cells. Shoelaces with intact plastic tips do not unravel and thus keep our shoes tied and our steps safe; similarly, for successful cell division, which is happening all the time in our bodies, we need the telomeres on the DNA to keep duplicating accurately, without errors called mutations, and working as well as possible.

Schematic of Chromosomes and Telomeres

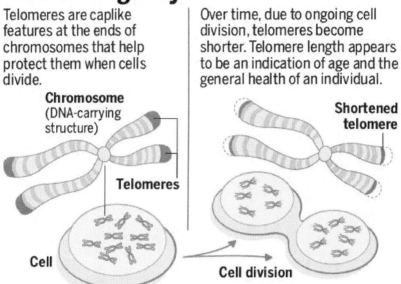

Source: The Nobel Committee for Physiology   ASSOCIATED PRESS

People with longer telomeres have lower death rates from cancers and many other diseases of later life. Long-term stress and negative thinking can prematurely shorten telomeres. Telomeres respond to what's going on in your life!

Blackburn and Epel provide evidence from their telomere research that regular exercise, a "Mediterranean-style" diet, good sleep habits, and taking measures to reduce the impact of chronic psychological stress are all associated with a slower rate of cellular aging. The authors also point to growing evidence that our early life experiences and social connections throughout life are important for successful ageing.

Telomeres get shorter as we age, but the rate at which this happens is influenced by a host of genetic and lifestyle factors, especially how much chronic stress presents in our lives and how we cope with that stress. Some 80-year-olds look and feel like 60-year-olds and some 60-year-olds appear more like 80-year-olds!

15. Stress

Stress is often described as a feeling of being overwhelmed, worried, or run-down. Stress can affect people of all ages, genders, and circumstances, and can lead to both physical and psychological health issues. By definition, **stress** is any uncomfortable emotional experience accompanied by predictable biochemical, physiological, and behavioral changes.

Stress hormones are released in times of perceived crisis regardless of age, marital status, income, or level of education. The characteristics of a stressful situation remain the same for everyone. The ingredients are always novelty, unpredictability, a threat to the self, and poor sense of control.

16. Acute Stress

Anything from everyday responsibilities like work and family to serious life events such as a new medical diagnosis, war, or the death of a loved one can trigger stress. For immediate, short-term situations, stress can be beneficial to your health. It can help you cope with potentially serious situations. Your body responds to stress by releasing hormones that increase your heart and breathing rates and ready your muscles to respond. It also primes the immune system for any potential wound or need to fight infection. Even non-dangerous situations and psychological pressures such as work deadlines, exams, and sporting events produce acute stress.

In your brain, the hypothalamus gets the ball rolling by telling your adrenal glands to release the stress hormones adrenaline and cortisol. These hormones rev up the heartbeat and send blood rushing to the areas that need it most in an emergency, such as your muscles, heart, brain, and other important organs. When the perceived fear is gone, the hypothalamus should tell all systems to go back to normal. The physical effects of acute stress usually do not last long and can be managed.

Managing stress begins with recognizing the signs that you are responding to a stressor. How? Listen to your body. When you feel your heart beginning to race, feel flushed, start to sweat, feel edgy and angry, you are likely having a stress response.

What can you do? The contexts in which we often experience stress do not always lend themselves to immediate management techniques. Starting to meditate or doing calisthenics or yoga in the middle of a stressful meeting may be inappropriate!

Some people find that repeating a mantra or mentally recalling a calming image is helpful. Quickly re-framing the issue may help. For example, the landlord wants to talk to you. Instead of immediately assuming that means a costly rent increase, perhaps he is sending a handyman to fix a leaky faucet. One should not automatically leap to fearful expectations. Slow down; it may or may not be what you are worrying about.

When we repeatedly release stress hormones, many systems, such as high blood pressure and high blood sugar, stay activated. These body systems do not fare well in constant alert mode and can start to break down. We are now dealing with chronic stress.

17. Chronic Stress

Chronic stress is the response to emotional pressure suffered for a prolonged period of time in which an individual perceives they have little or no control. Many scientists think that our stress response system was not designed to be constantly activated. This overuse may contribute to the breakdown of many bodily systems. In fact, chronic stress has been linked to heart disease, high blood pressure, high cholesterol, type II diabetes, and cancer. Psychologically, chronic stress also causes wear and tear in the form of increased anxiety, depression, and burnout.

The effects of chronic stress are worse for people already at risk for developing these and other problems. For instance, if one has a family history of heart disease, diabetes, high blood pressure, or has unhealthy lifestyle habits, then chronic stress can flip the switch that turns on these health problems.

Chronic stress is also a factor in behaviors such as overeating or not eating enough, alcohol or drug abuse, and social withdrawal.

Some potential causes of chronic stress in older people include: Loss of beloved spouse or close friend whom one spent much time with, living with a serious illness with a poor prognosis, possibly painful and limiting mobility, great financial difficulty, long-term care of ill close family members, living in a dangerous neighborhood (a war zone would be the extreme form of that), being involved in an abusive relationship, or inability to resolve arguments with close family, especially spouse or children.

18. Major Depression

Worldwide, depression will be the single biggest cause of disability in the next 20 years. However, treatment for it has not changed much in the last three decades. Almost all of the antidepressant medications have similar mechanisms of action: facilitating communication between neurons in brain synapses. When this treatment doesn't work, and it doesn't work about half the time, and psychotherapy also fails, patients are in trouble.

Recently, University of Cambridge Professor Edward Bullimore published a book[32] summarizing some of the new science on the link between depression and inflammation of the body and brain. He explains that we now strongly suspect that mental disorders can have their root cause in an overactive immune system. The book outlines a future in which treatments could be specifically targeted to break the vicious cycle of stress, inflammation, and depression. The "Inflamed Mind" suggests a new way of looking at how mind, brain, and body all work together in a sometimes-misguided effort to help us survive in a hostile world. It offers insights into how we can approach depression and other mental disorders more effectively in the future.

For years, it has been known that inflammatory markers are particularly increased in patients with resistant depression. Also, inflammatory stimuli utilized in the treatment of other illnesses, such as interleukins for cancer treatment, are known to cause significant depressive symptoms.

As Professor Bullimore says, "The immune system is talking to your brain." So, where does chronic inflammation come from? One place is from chronic stress. Chronic infection and obesity are also drivers of chronic inflammation. Other possibilities are disruptions in the microbiome in the gut and elsewhere. Thus, inflammatory signals are coming to the brain from the body's periphery.

In chronic stress, neurons become excited along with the brain's own immune system. Cytokines are produced, which draw inflammatory cells from the peripheral blood. At the same time, the blood-brain barrier becomes permeable, and inflammatory cells, such as monocytes and macrophages, become more prevalent in the brain. The inflammatory process makes synaptic transmission less responsive and more excitable. All of this results in decreasing brain cell growth factors like BDNF.

Almost every significant medical illness involves inflammation. That includes not only those illnesses involving external pathogens such as viruses and bacteria, but immune-related diseases such as cancer and autoimmune diseases. In addition, chronic inflammation seems to play an important role in metabolic illnesses, such as diabetes, cardiovascular disease, and morbid obesity.

Cortisol, first and foremost, maintains energy balance. When we expend energy by using up calories, our body needs to replace the lost energy. Cortisol carries the message: refuel.

So, the brain and cortisol are always trying to protect us. Unfortunately, when we are chronically stressed, they will "help us out" by increasing appetite and storing this extra energy in the form of fat tissue. The end result is truncal obesity or fat around our midsection.

Our brains have not changed much since we were hunter-gathers chasing mammoths, so we react similarly to the stressors of the modern world.

The stress response system and its end-product, cortisol, are key players. When the cortisol system becomes deregulated, as in reacting to continuing stress, it affects all other systems that depend on its integrity to function.

19. Chronic Stress and Cardiovascular Disease

Chronic stress is also associated with an increased risk of cardiovascular disease This risk is on par with that of other major cardiovascular risk factors such as obesity, smoking, and high cholesterol.

Stress prompts activation of both the sympathetic nervous system and the hypothalamic–pituitary–adrenal axis. Heart rate and blood pressure increase contributing to the dysfunction of the cells that line the inside of blood vessels. However, this mechanism does not entirely explain the link between stress and cardiovascular disease.

Tawakol and his associates[33] recently showed that resting metabolic activity within the amygdala, a key component of the brain's network involved in stress, significantly predicts the development of cardiovascular disease independently of established cardiovascular risk factors. Amygdala activity was associated with increased manufacture of immune blood cells and increased arterial inflammation.

These findings provide new and important insights, specifically that the amygdala could be a key structure in the mechanism linking stress to cardiovascular events, and that increased regulation of blood tissues may have some effect on the brain-cardiovascular relationship.

Activation of the brain stress network and its downstream consequences, including the formation of blood cells and increased arterial inflammation, could be targets for therapies designed to interrupt a vicious cycle between stress and cardiovascular events. For example, meditation has been shown to reduce amygdala activity. In a study of 226 individuals, 42 of those randomly assigned to a 12-week stress-reduction course experienced an approximately 50 percent reduction in cardiovascular disease events compared with individuals who underwent cardiac rehabilitation but not stress management training.

So, if chronic stress is so pervasive and so destructive to many of our most important organs including the immune system, brain and heart, why does not everybody suffer these diseases? Do people vary in their capacity to deal with stress, even chronic stress?

Are some individuals more resilient than others, and how does that come about?

20. Emotional Resilience

Resilience is defined as adapting well in the face of adversity, trauma, tragedy, threats or other significant sources of stress, such as family and relationship problems, serious health problems, or financial stressors. It addresses the ability to successfully overcome difficult experiences and stay calm in the face of anticipated trouble.

Emotional pain, anxiety, and sadness are common in people whenever one suffers major adversity or trauma in their lives. Fortunately, everyone has some resiliency and can cope with some problems. It can be seen as the individual's built-in as well as learned methods to problem-solve. It's part of being human and alive. Likely, cows and other animals are calmer and happier than most humans! The difference lies in part in the human's ability to hold complex thoughts and feelings inside and visualize future possibilities for good or bad. That processing is likely to involve considerable emotional distress.

Resilience is not like an on/off switch, or a trait that people either have or do not have. Rather it involves a continuum of helpful behaviors, thoughts, and actions that can be learned and developed in anyone.

Developing resilience is a personal journey. Not only do you start off with an inherited emotional temperament which is unique, but we all have different life experiences.

One place where resiliency starts is early infancy and childhood. These early years are crucial in developing the emotional resiliency that will sustain individuals throughout life. That early bonding is not all that goes into creating a resilient individual, even through age 80 and beyond, but it is the best-researched phenomena, and we will now look into that in some detail.

In 1992, a developmental psychologist named Emmy Werner wrote a book[34] discussing the results of a thirty-two-year long-term project. She had followed a group of six hundred and ninety-eight children, in Kauai, Hawaii, from before birth through their third decade of life. Along the way, she monitored them for any exposure[35] to stress: maternal stress in utero, poverty, problems in the family, and so on. Two-thirds of the children came from backgrounds that were essentially stable, successful, and happy; the other third qualified as "at risk." They had four or more risk factors by age two.

She discovered that not all of the at-risk children reacted to stress in the same way. Two-thirds of them "developed serious learning or behavior problems by the age of ten, or had delinquency records, mental health problems, or teenage pregnancies by the age of eighteen." But the remaining third developed into "competent, confident, and caring young adults." They had attained academic, domestic, and social success. They grew up to be adults who "loved well, worked well, played well, and expected well."

Werner found that several elements predicted resilience. Some elements had to do with luck: a resilient child might have a strong bond with a supportive caregiver, parent, teacher, or other mentor-like figure. But another, quite large set of elements, were psychological. These concerned how resilient children responded to the environment. From a young age, resilient children tended to "meet the world on their own terms." They were autonomous and independent, would seek out new experiences, and had a "positive social orientation." "Though not especially gifted, these children used whatever skills they had effectively," Werner wrote.

Perhaps most importantly, the resilient children had what psychologists call an "internal locus of control": they believed that they, and not their circumstances, affected their achievements. The resilient children saw themselves as the orchestrators of their own fates. In fact, on a scale that measured locus of control, they scored more than two standard deviations away from the rest of the group. Werner also discovered that resilience could change over time. Some resilient children were especially unlucky: they experienced multiple strong stressors at vulnerable points, and their resilience evaporated.

In order to understand more about resilience and how it helps people of all ages deal with chronic stress, we need to start at the very beginning. Infants could not be more helpless and fragile. What keeps an infant alive? Is it just breast milk, or is more going on? Is there is a more helpless and stressful situation than being a hungry newborn? How does an infant cope with that and other stresses?

Are some mothers better than others at reassuring their infants and children? Does that influence an individual's ability to cope with stress throughout life, even past 80? What about mothers who are not good at that task or children raised in an orphanage?

21. The Monkey's Mothering Attachment

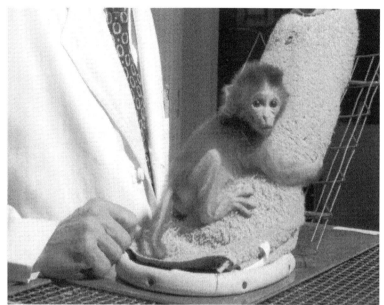

Harlow's Infant Monkey with Soft Mother Surrogate

Harry Harlow's empirical work with primates is now considered a "classic" in behavioral science, revolutionizing our understanding of the role that social relationships play in early development. In the 1950s and 60s, psychological research in the United States was dominated by behaviorists and psychoanalysts, who supported the view that babies became attached to their mothers because they provided food. Harlow and other social and cognitive psychologists argued that this perspective overlooked the importance of comfort, companionship, and love in promoting healthy development.

Using isolation and maternal deprivation, Harlow showed the impact of contact comfort on primate development. Infant rhesus monkeys were taken away from their mothers and raised in a laboratory setting, with some infants placed in separate cages away from peers. In social isolation, the monkeys showed disturbed behavior, staring blankly, circling their cages, and engaging in self-mutilation. When the isolated infants were re-introduced to the group, many stayed separate from the group, and some even died after refusing to eat.

Even with partial isolation, infants showed reclusive tendencies, including clinging to their cloth diapers. Harlow speculated that the soft material may simulate the comfort provided by a mother's touch. Based on this observation, Harlow designed his now-famous surrogate mother experiment.

In this study, Harlow took infant monkeys from their biological mothers and gave them two inanimate surrogates (i.e. mother substitutes): one was a simple construction of wire and wood, and the second was covered in foam rubber and soft terry cloth. The infants were assigned to one of two conditions. In the first, the wire mother had a milk bottle and the cloth mother did not; in the second, the cloth mother had the food while the wire mother had none.

In both conditions, Harlow found that the infant monkeys spent significantly more time with the terry cloth mother than they did with the wire mother. When only the wire mother had food, the babies came to the wire mother to feed and immediately returned to cling to the cloth surrogate.

When placed in a novel environment with a surrogate mother, infant monkeys would explore the area, run back to the surrogate mother when startled, and then venture out to explore again. Without a surrogate mother, the infants were paralyzed with fear, huddled in a ball sucking their thumbs. If an alarming noise-making toy was placed in the cage, an infant with a surrogate mother present would explore and attack the toy; without a surrogate mother, the infant would cower in fear.

Together, these studies produced empirical evidence for the primacy of the parent-child attachment relationship and the importance of maternal touch in infant development.

Harlow also demonstrated the importance of contact with peers. The maternally deprived young monkeys were able to learn from their properly raised peers.[36]

22. Human Attachment

John Bowlby (1907-1990), a British child psychiatrist and psychoanalyst known for his "attachment theory" knew of Harlow's work with monkeys. He went on to show that human infants and children were also adversely affected by maternal deprivation.

He defined attachment as a long-lasting psychological connection with a meaningful person that causes pleasure and soothes in times of stress.

Bowlby's research focused on child delinquents and hospitalized children. These studies documented the negative effects of maternal deprivation on human babies. Development suffered when the mother was either non-responsive or absent for long spans of time within the child's first two years of life. Bowlby believed that children have an innate need to develop a close relationship with one main figure, usually the mother. When this does not occur, there are negative consequences for child development. These children subsequently showed lower intelligence and a predisposition to depression, aggression, delinquency, and psychopathy.

23. Maternal Deprivation

Research into Maternal Deprivation also turned to orphan studies as a means of studying the effects of deprivation. An opportunity to look at the effects of deprivation and institutionalization arose in Romania in the 1990s. The former president of Romania, Nicolai Ceaucescu, ordered Romanian women to have five children. Many Romanian parents couldn't afford to keep the children, and many ended up in orphanages.

Rutter and associates (2011) followed a group of 165 Romanian orphans adopted in Britain to test to what extent good care could make up for poor early experiences in institutions. Physical, cognitive, and emotional development was assessed at 4, 6, 11, and 15 years of age. A group of 15 English children adopted around the same time served as a control group.

When they first arrived in the UK, half the adoptees showed signs of mental retardation and were undernourished. At the age of 11, the children showed differential rates of recovery that were linked to their age of adoption; those adopted before they were 6 months old did much better than later adoptees.[37]

24. Chronic Stress versus Emotional Resilience

Stressors can be so intense that resilience is overwhelmed. Most people, in short, have a breaking point. However, the reverse is true as well. People who weren't resilient earlier (possibly in childhood) may learn the requisite skills over time. Even in old age, damage from early privation versus positive learning may be playing out.

Beyond recognizing resilience as "achieving a positive outcome in the face of adversity," the flexibility of the brain based upon healthy architecture emerges as a primary consideration. We have seen that brain architecture continues to show plasticity throughout adult life, and studies of gene expression and epigenetic regulation reveal a dynamic and ever-changing brain.

Reactivation of plasticity in individuals lacking emotional resilience is a new challenge for research. Our old friends, physical activity, mental stimulation, adequate sleep, social support, finding meaning in life, mindful meditation, and yoga are emerging as helpful. The search is also on for pharmaceutical agents that can help.

25. Characteristics of Resilient Individuals

How do adults who experience chronic stress survive, manage, and thrive, and what resources enable them to do so?

The scientific literature suggests the following resources and characteristics are helpful. They may have been learned from parental figures or from other role models. A long life offers the opportunity to continue to learn what helps get through difficulty and what does not. We continue to learn.

The list includes relatively objective characteristics of the individual such as physical strength, good health, and high intelligence, as well as more subjective things such as perceived mastery over the environment or perceived support.

Strong marriages, good friendships, cohesive families and belonging to a community are also important. The individual may become stronger over time as a function of successfully confronting stressors. This process continues throughout life, as much in the 80s and 90s as in earlier years.

That is all very encouraging, but what about non-resilient individuals? What happens to them? Are there any examples of that?

26. A Third-World Mental Hospital

My career in psychiatry began before I was a psychiatrist. I was in charge of the medical and psychiatric care of 300 older female inmates at a Panamanian mental hospital (1964-65) before I started my residency training at Harvard/Mass Mental Health Center in 1966. I had come to Panama as the staff physician for the Peace Corps. Maintaining the health of 250 American volunteers was my formal job. However, I had some extra time available and asked the Panamanian Minister of Health where I might volunteer my services. The minister suggested Mattias Hernandez, the large government mental hospital located on the outskirts of Panama City.

When I arrived at Mattias Hernandez, I entered the grounds through a guarded gate. It proved to be the only entrance to a very run down five-acre complex totally enclosed by a high concrete wall. At the time, this psychiatric institution had approximately 1,600 patients distributed in six courtyards. Males and females were housed separately. A few patients were out and about doing trash pick-up or painting concrete benches. However, they were very much the exception.

Within a day, I found myself in charge of all the chronically ill, mostly older female patients who lived in one of the courtyards. None of the staff psychiatrists ever visited, even once. All the patients looked more like animals than human beings. They presented with scarred faces and limbs, dirty, disheveled and ripped clothing, or none at all. They all had the same blank stare, and most barely communicated verbally. Even then, what phrases they did get out usually made little or no sense.

The courtyard consisted of numerous concrete benches, a large drainage ditch, and the ground floor of a multistory building whose upper floors had collapsed. What remained of the building was used as a cafeteria during the daytime and a dormitory at night. There were not enough beds for all the patients and no mattresses at all. In one corner of the courtyard, which I never visited, I was told there was some tap water, a hose for showering, and some rudimentary toilets. Patients ate food from a trough, similar to how animals are fed. Judging from the amount of diarrhea and other intestinal complaints and the results of occasional stool cultures, the food was contaminated with amoebas and other tropical parasites. Most of the patients spent their time fighting with one another, coming to blows over a bit of food, a shred of clothing, a shady spot, etc. Screaming, moaning, praying, and bickering were ever-present sounds. Most patients paced the grounds in a haphazard way. Open sex was the norm, whether masturbation, between two individuals, or just a group orgy. Anything went!

One nurse was on duty to hand out medications and to do first aid. She never left the office, nor did any of the other professional staff leave the safety of the office. We communicated only through a locked half door with the patient courtyard. During the day, there might be an aide available to go into the courtyard to help break up fights between patients. Besides me, there was one other physician, a female intern just out of medical school, who had responsibilities throughout the rest of the hospital as well. I was there most afternoons, three days per week, when I wasn't out of town.

Any patients needing medical help would be brought into the nurses' office, where the intern or I would treat and bandage open wounds to prevent infection or immobilize broken bones. Lacking any psychiatric training, we mostly prescribed anti-seizure medications, antibiotics, and drugs to treat parasitic infections. The few antipsychotics pills we could get from the hospital pharmacy were mostly reserved for acutely agitated patients.

Even the ritual of handing out the medicines was bizarre. My favorite patient, who at least knew I was an American, would come by to warn the others that they were "loco" to trust pills prescribed by a "gringo, so-called doctor."

Almost all the patients had been in this facility fifteen years or more. From what I could gather from the primitive records, 70 patients had come in diagnosed only with epilepsy. The rest were thought to be psychotic. After a time, everyone was crazy, whether they started out that way or not. The place looked like and smelled like a filthy zoo. I decided that it was as close to Hell as I could imagine. Only the flames and odor of sulfur were missing!

The intern and I wanted to do something but felt overwhelmed by the sheer number of regressed patients and the stench of the courtyard. We finally decided to set up a new small unit to try to salvage at least a small number of patients. The intern proved to be an extremely effective solicitor of donations from the business community. In short order, she arranged for fifteen cots with mattresses, basic clothing, towels, radios, clocks, a television, and even combs and cosmetics for our carefully selected patients. We put all of these things into a freshly painted former storage area adjacent to the nursing station. Best of all, we arranged for food service from the employee cafeteria instead of the usual patient gruel.

After pouring through the rudimentary patient records, interviewing staff, and soliciting volunteers from appropriate patients, we introduced fifteen patients from the courtyard to the new medical unit. Not only would they have a safe place to sleep and eat, but they would also be allowed out of the unit into the hospital grounds during the daytime. The plan was to gradually re-civilize them and see if we could get any ready for discharge. As a first step, we did blood counts, urinalyses, and examined stool for parasites. In addition to treating anemia, urinary tract infections, and parasites like amoebas, hookworm, and digestive tract round worm infections, we boosted anti-epileptic drugs like Dilantin and Phenobarbital to levels where they actually controlled seizures in patients with epilepsy. We also raised the dose of antipsychotic medication to levels that began to stop delusions, hallucinations, and other psychotic features in most of the patients.

What happened next truly astonished me and probably accounts for my subsequent decision to change my career path from internal medicine to psychiatry. After a few weeks, we were able to discharge one patient after much detective work on the intern's part to find her family. However, that was our only success. That, too, was short-lived as the patient returned after a few days, dropped off by her family in the middle of the night. The patient wouldn't talk about it afterwards, only to say that there was no place for her in the family after all these years.

All the other patients, with tears in their eyes, would approach us one-by-one, every week or so to say that they wanted to return to the courtyard. They felt free there. The new surroundings demanded too much of them. They did not feel like going to sleep when the lights went out, eating at set times, or sitting quietly while watching television. There was no place to roam freely, discharge their anger with a good fistfight, or just piss where they wanted to. They cried because they knew that both the intern and I had put a lot of energy and hope into them, but they were lost causes. They had no family who cared about them, hadn't talked to anyone on the outside in years, and had too much confusion in their heads to ever make it back to a society that they only remembered vaguely. All of their friends were in the courtyard, and they did not have to behave there. It was something they had now gotten used to and missed, despite the danger and chaos. To behave was too hard, to think of ever getting out of Mattias Hernandez was frightening, and they no longer had any expectations. Nor was what they remembered of their prior life hopeful. Most had been abjectly poor, rejected by their families and communities for their strange behavior, and had always been made fun of.

Usually, we were able to talk the patients into staying a few days or weeks longer in the special unit, but still they kept beseeching us to leave, until finally we would cave in and allow them back into the courtyard. Replacements fared the same way. Perhaps a total of 30 patients tried our program, some for several months, but all eventually wanted back into the courtyard.

At the time, I was mostly numb and puzzled by the experience. I dreaded going back to the hospital, but nonetheless always showed up. I had promised to work there, was needed, and also didn't want to desert the intern who had so dutifully followed my lead in our failed program.

Fortunately, the rest of my year in Panama was quite successful in that I became gradually more proficient in Spanish and easily able to handle my duties as a general physician for the mostly quite healthy volunteers.

My time at Mattias Hernandez came to an end when I accepted a promotion to spend my second year on the Peace Corps staff in Washington, DC. The moment I fastened my seat belt for the flight out of Panama marked a sudden easing of the rumbling and dull pain in my stomach that accompanied an unwanted 20-pound weight loss. It certainly was not Panama in general, as my wife, whom I met later, grew up in Panama, and we returned happily to visit her family for many years. It wasn't the Peace Corps either, as I served the next year happily and healthfully in Washington without a twitch of stomach pain or loss of appetite.

To this day, I am not entirely sure why we were so unsuccessful, but unsuccessful we were, and it was that humility and experience that brought me into psychiatry. Later on, I heard that the intern left the country for a child psychiatry residency in Argentina.

Perhaps institutionalization and chronic mental illness, allowed to fester, particularly in older, non-resilient individuals, is untreatable. If you ever think your situation is untenable and the worst that anyone can be in, I would advise thinking of the patients at Mattias Hernandez. Being poor, old, and crazy in a 3rd world country, at least in the 1960's, was not pleasant end of life.

27. Are the Old Happier than the Young?

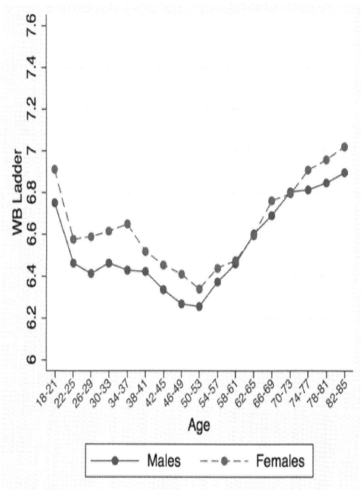

Wellbeing as Reported by Age

In 2008, the Gallup Organization conducted a telephone survey of over 340,000 individuals in the United States, allowing a determination of Wellbeing (WB) by age.

Whatever definition of WB one assesses, either in men or women, older persons are not less happy. Quite to the contrary, older persons are clearly happier with their lives than most other age groups. Only those between 18-21 years of age come close. Reasons for the age patterns of WB were not explicitly hypothesized, but several variables could plausibly contribute to the increase in WB over age. For example, it is plausible that WB improves when children leave home, reducing levels of family conflict and financial burden.

A recent article[38] by Judith Graham published in the Washington Post does a good job of explaining and personalizing the phenomenon of older individuals continuing to feel positive about their well-being in the face of obvious objective deterioration in their health and capacities. We quote extensively from this short piece of journalistic research.

Data from the 2017 National Health Interview Survey, administered by the Centers for Disease Control and Prevention, tell us something about why older individuals feel positive about their lives and prospects.

When asked to rate their overall health, adults aged 65 to 74 described it as excellent (18 percent), very good (32 percent), or good (32 percent). Only 18 percent of this age group had a negative perspective, describing their health as fair (14 percent) or poor (4 percent).

This trend toward positivity is also evident among adults age 75 and older. They rated their health as excellent (12 percent), very good (28 percent), or good (33 percent), while only 27 percent gave a fair (20 percent) or poor (7 percent) evaluation.

This perception of well-being flies in the face of the fact that 60 percent of older adults have two or more chronic illnesses, such as diabetes, arthritis, hypertension, heart disease, or kidney disease, and much higher rates of physical impairment than other age groups.

However, just as chronic stress in the form of medical problems intensifies, the survivors are resilient individuals who have adapted and changed their attitudes and expectations as they have aged.

Older adults think differently about their health. The components of health they tend to value are vitality, emotional well-being, social relationships, and remaining active and satisfied with life. Poor physical health plays a less important role.

"Being healthy means being able to continue doing what I like: going to the theater, organizing programs, enjoying the arts, walking," said Lorelei Goldman, 80, of Evanston, Ill., who has had ovarian and breast cancer. She also describes her health as "good."

"I have all my faculties and good, longtime friendships," Goldman said. "I used to be a bad sleeper, but now I'm sleeping much better. Almost every day, there are moments of clarity and joy. I'm involved in a lot of activities that are sustaining."

Even when older adults are coping with medical conditions and impairments, they can usually think of people their age who are worse off — those who have died or gone to nursing homes, said Ellen Idler, a professor of sociology at Emory University in Atlanta and a leading researcher in the field of "self-rated health." By comparison, seniors still able to live on their own may feel "I'm doing pretty well."

At some point, merely surviving can be interpreted as a sign of good health. "People hit their 80s and 90s, look around, and feel pretty good about just being alive," Idler said.

That isn't true for younger adults, who measure their health against an ideal "there shouldn't be anything wrong with me" standard. Obviously, expectations for what constitutes good health change as people move into later life.

"Older people expect some deterioration in health and aren't thrown off course in the same way when it occurs," said Jason Schnittker, a professor of sociology at the University of Pennsylvania who has studied self-rated health.

Resilience is also at play. As older adults adapt to illness and other physical changes, they tend to adjust their outlook. "I may be handicapped, but I can still walk," one 86-year-old woman told Swiss researchers after being hospitalized from a fall and forced to use a stick to get around. She considered herself fortunate and rated her health positively. "As long as you can get to church, as long as you can walk, you can say all's well," a man in his 80s declared after becoming severely disabled because of a slipped disk in his spine and an embolism. He, too, felt good about his health.

Lest you think older adults' bias toward positivity is a sign of denial or a lack of objectivity, a large body of research shows it's highly meaningful. "Self-rated health is very strongly predictive of longevity," as well as other outcomes, such as cognitive health and use of health-care services, Schnittker said.

This positivity isn't universal. African Americans, Hispanics, people with lower levels of income and education, and individuals with poor social connections are more likely to rate their health negatively as they age. At younger ages, women rate their health more poorly than men, but this changes in later life, with men becoming more likely to report worse health and women becoming more optimistic.

For example, an older person has severe arthritis and systemic lupus erythematosus (a serious auto-immune disease). Nonetheless, she considers her health "very good" and credits her optimism, close relationships, and "extremely active life." Poor health would mean being bedridden, "not being able to go out or be as mobile as I am, or extended suffering," she said. "My attitude now is I've lived 70 good years, and I hope the next years are rich as well." "I think most people fear old age, but once they get there, it's like, 'Oh, I'm still going, I'm still okay.' And fear becomes acceptance."

28. The Future: Longevity and Anti-Aging Research

Research into longevity and healthy aging has progressed rapidly in recent years, but intense interest from the public, corporations, and the media has created an environment in which unfounded claims can be hard to separate from scientific facts.

In February 2019, a group of 16 researchers from Harvard, MIT, and other institutions around the U.S. and Europe launched the nonprofit Academy for Health and Lifespan Research to promote future work, ease collaborations between scientists, and ensure that governments and corporations are making decisions based on the latest facts instead of rumor, speculation, or hype.[39]

In a new book,[40] Harvard Medical School Genetics Professor David Sinclair explains how science has moved from being able to extend health and lifespan of simple organisms like yeast and worms and flies to being able to do this quite easily in animals, in mice, and monkeys. Instead of tackling one chronic disease at a time, he believes we can develop medicines that will treat aging at its source and thereby have a much greater impact on health and lifespan than drugs that target a single disease.

In a chapter entitled, "A Better Pill to Swallow," Sinclair goes on to describe the science and history behind the first of these potential medicines. He details the experimental data for rapamycin, resveratrol, metformin, and NAD (Nicotinamide Adenine Nucleotide) boosters to extend life and decrease the incidence of chronic diseases.

None of these molecules has yet gained FDA approval for this purpose. They all seem to work by stabilizing the genome and epigenome which otherwise show increasing disorganization with age across all of species of plant and animal.

We now conclude our overview of how to lead a healthier and possibly longer life. We hope you follow our advice. It is also not the last word. Please continue to learn, for example by reading the David Sinclair book referenced above. Who knows what the next development in this exciting field will be?

About the Authors

Wolfgang Berg

Born in Bremen, Germany, Wolfgang Berg studied macroeconomics in Freiburg, Germany and graduated with a business administration degree from the University of Munich, Germany.

After ten years as product manager, marketing manager, and CEO of a large multinational consumer products corporation, he started his own market research and consulting company in the USA. That company eventually became a small, market-leading electronics and sports optics manufacturer.

His work led him to countries all over Europe, North and South America, and Japan. In each place, he conducted consumer research, often in focus groups, exploring behavior and attitudes of consumers. He developed marketing plans, products, and a variety of businesses.

His hobbies are sailing and scuba diving, about which he wrote nine books. He also has been, and still is, a nationally ranked tennis player. In addition, he has climbed and skied all over the Alps. At age 80, he sailed solo 2,200 miles and did a rock climb of five hours. And at age 82, he won the consolation round of the tennis world championship in the 80-year-old category.

Jay M. Pomerantz, M.D.

Dr. Pomerantz received an A.B. from Hamilton College and an M.D. from Yale University School of Medicine. Following a rotating internship at the Hospital of the University of Pennsylvania, he served in the US Peace Corps, first as a staff physician in Panama and later as Medical Director for Latin America. He then completed a residency in psychiatry at Massachusetts Mental Health Center and a fellowship in Community Mental Health at Harvard Medical School. After that, he moved to western Massachusetts as Regional Administrator for the Massachusetts Department of Mental Health. After 7 years at that position, Dr. Pomerantz spent the next 43 years in private practice. His awards include being a "Distinguished Life Fellow" of the American Psychiatric Association and winner of the "Outstanding Psychiatrist Award" of the Massachusetts Psychiatric Association in 2000 for the "Advancement of the Profession."

Since retiring from psychiatric practice in 2015, Dr. Pomerantz has been teaching at Temple University's Osher Lifelong Learning Institute (OLLI). Among the courses he has taught are "Neuroscience of Memory," "Genes and Stem Cells," "Immunological Approach to Cancer Treatment," and "Modern Psychiatry: More Neuroscience and Less Freud."

End Notes

[1] https://www.itftennis.com/news/307287.aspx

[2] Roberson NA, Hillary RF, McCartney DL et al. Age related haemopoiesis is associated with increased epigenetic age. Current Biology. 19 August 2019; 786-787.

[3] A person's biological age can lag behind or exceed chronological age. It is measured in a variety of ways including how many chemical modifications, such as methyl groups tag DNA. The pattern of these tags changes during the course of a lifetime.

[4] Kaluza J, Håkansson N, Harris HR, et al. Influence of anti-inflammatory diet and smoking on mortality and survival in men and women: two prospective cohort studies. Journal of Internal Medicine, 2018; DOI: 10.1111/joim.12823

[5] Fleg JL, Morrell CH, Bos AG, Brant LJ, Talbot LA, Wright JG, Lakatta EG. Accelerated longitudinal decline of aerobic capacity in healthy older adults. Circulation 112:674-682, 2005.

[6] Fleg JL, Schulman S, O'Connor FC, Gerstenblith G, Becker LC, Fortney S, Goldberg AP, Lakatta EG. Cardiovascular responses to exhaustive upright cycle exercise in highly trained older men. J Appl Physiol 77:1500-1506, 1994.

[7] Booth LN, Brunet A. The aging genome. Mol Cell (2016);62(5): 728-744

[8] AARP Bulletin July/August 2019 Vol 60 page 6

[9] https://www.health.harvard.edu/blog/is-red-wine-good-actually-for-your-heart-2018021913285

[10] https://www.nbcnews.com/better/health/smiling-can-trick-your-brain-happiness-boost-your-health-ncna822591

[11] https://easylivingfl.com/leading-causes-death-65-year-olds/

[12] https://www.cdc.gov/flu/spotlights/2016-2017/vaccine-reduces-severe-outcomes.htm?CDC_AA_refVal=https%3A%2F%2Fwww.cdc.gov%2Ffl u%2Fspotlights%2Fvaccine-reduces-severe-outcomes.htm

[13] Sei J. Lee, Alan S. Go, Karla Lindquist, Daniel Bertenthal, Kenneth E. Covinsky.Am J Public Health. 2008 Jul; 98(7): 1209–1214.

[14] Paul CA, Au R., Fredman L et al. Association of alcohol consumption with brain volume in Framigham study.Arch Neurol. 2008;65(10):1363-1367

[15] Sabia S, Elbaz A, Britton A. et all. Alcohol consumption and cognitive decline in early old age. Neurology 2014;82:332-339

[16] Lipoff JB. Don't fear the reaper. JAMA 2019;322:929-930

[17] E. Kandel. In search of memory W.W. Norton Co.; New York, 2006

[18] Maguire EA, Gadian DG, Johnsrude IS, et al. Navigation-related structural change in the hippocampi of taxi drivers. Proc Natl Acad Sci U S A. 2000;97(8):4398–4403. doi:10.1073/pnas.070039597

[19] Pauwels L, Chalavi S, Swinnen SP. Aging and brain plasticity. 2018 Aging (Albany NY). 10(8):1789–1790. doi:10.18632/aging.101514

[20] Cui, Z., Feng R., Jacobs S., Duan Y., Wang H., Cao X., et al. (2013). Increased NR2A:NR2B ratio compresses long-term depression range and constrains long-term memory.

[21] Verghese J, Lipton RB, Katz MJ, et al. Leisure activities and the risk of dementia in the elderly. N Engl J Med. 2003;348:2508–2516.

[22] Wilson RS, Mendes De Leon CF, Barnes LL, et al. Participation in cognitively stimulating activities and risk of incident Alzheimer disease. JAMA. 2002;287:742–748

[23] Fritsch T, Smyth KA, Debanne SM, Petot GJ, Friedland RP. Participation in novelty-seeking leisure activities and Alzheimer's

disease. Journal of Geriatric Psychiatry and Neurology. 2005;18:134–141.

[24] William E Reichman; Alexandra J Fiocco; Nathan S Rose. Exercising the Brain to Avoid Cognitive Decline: Examining the Evidence. .Aging Health. 2010;6(5):565-584.

[25] A Snowdon, David. (2003). Healthy Aging and Dementia: Findings from the Nun Study. Annals of internal medicine. 139. 450-4. 10.7326/0003-4819-139

[26] Healthy Brain, Happy Life (2015) by Wendy Suzuki, Ph.D

[27] David A. Raichlen[1,] et al. Front. Hum. Neurosci., 29 November 2016 | https://doi.org/10.3389/fnhum.2016.00610

[28] This section owes much (including the cartoon to Michael Dregni's summary article on the topic (2018) https://experiencelife.com/article/this-is-your-brain-on-exercise/

[29] Karsenty G et al. Gpr158 mediates osteocalcin's regulation of cognition. Journal of Experimental Medicine, August 2017 DOI: 10.1084/jem.20171320

[30] https://www.researchgate.net/blog/post/cleaning-while-we-sleep-a-novel-approach-in-alzheimers-research

[31] https://www.researchgate.net/blog/post/cleaning-while-we-sleep-a-novel-approach-in-alzheimers-research

[32] Edward Bullimore (2018). The Inflamed Mind

[33] Tawakol A, Ishai A, Takx R AP, et al. Relation between resting amygdalar activity and cardiovascular events: a longitudinal and cohort study. Lancet 2017;389:834-45.

[34] Overcoming the Odds: High Risk Children from Birth to Adulthood (Werner & Smith, 1992)

[35] Overcoming the Odds: High Risk Children from Birth to Adulthood (Werner & Smith, 1992)

[36] Harlow H. F., Dodsworth R. O., & Harlow M. K. (1965). Total social isolation in monkeys. Proceedings of the National Academy of Sciences of the United States of America. Retrieved from https://www.ncbi.nlm.nih.gov/pmc/articles/PMC285801/pdf/pnas00159-0105.pdf

[37] https://psychologyhub.co.uk/bowlbys-theory-of-maternal-deprivation-romanian-orphan-studies-effects-of-institutionalisation/

[38] Many older adults feel positive about their health. Here's why. Judith Graham, Washington Post. June 29, 2019

[39] https://news.harvard.edu/gazette/story/2019/03/anti-aging-research-prime-time-for-an-impact-on-the-globe/

[40] D. Sinclair. Lifespan, Why We Age—and Why We Don't Have To. (2019) Atria Books

Made in the USA
Lexington, KY
16 December 2019